Choice and Efficiency in Food Safety Policy

AEI STUDIES IN AGRICULTURAL POLICY

AGRICULTURAL POLICY REFORM IN THE UNITED STATES
Daniel A. Sumner, ed.

AGRICULTURAL TRADE POLICY: LETTING MARKETS WORK
Daniel A. Sumner

ASSESSING THE ENVIRONMENTAL IMPACT OF FARM POLICIES
Walter N. Thurman

CHOICE AND EFFICIENCY IN FOOD SAFETY POLICY
John M. Antle

THE ECONOMICS OF CROP INSURANCE AND DISASTER AID
Barry K. Goodwin and Vincent H. Smith

THE EFFECTS OF CREDIT POLICIES ON U.S. AGRICULTURE
Peter J. Barry

MAKING SCIENCE PAY: THE ECONOMICS OF AGRICULTURAL
R&D POLICY
Julian M. Alston and Philip G. Pardey

REFORMING AGRICULTURAL COMMODITY POLICY
Brian D. Wright and Bruce L. Gardner

Choice and Efficiency in Food Safety Policy

John M. Antle

The AEI Press

Publisher for the American Enterprise Institute

WASHINGTON, D.C.

1995

Available in the United States from the AEI Press, c/o Publisher Resources Inc., 1224 Heil Quaker Blvd., P.O. Box 7001, La Vergne, TN 37086-7001. Distributed outside the United States by arrangement with Eurospan, 3 Henrietta Street, London WC2E 8LU England.

Library of Congress Cataloging-in-Publication Data
Antle, John M.
    Choice and efficiency in food safety policy / John M. Antle.
      p. cm.—(AEI studies in agricultural policy)
    Includes bibliographical references
    ISBN 0-8447-3902-2 (cloth : alk. paper).
    1. Food adulturation and inspection. 2. Food—Quality.
    3. Food contamination. I. Title. II. Series
    TX531.A58   1995
    363.19′26—dc20   95-15001
                                                     CIP

1 3 5 7 9 10 8 6 4 2

The AEI PRESS
Publisher for the American Enterprise Institute
1150 17th Street, N.W., Washington, D.C. 20036

Printed in the United States of America

Contents

FOREWORD   *Christopher DeMuth*   vii

1 INTRODUCTION   1
  Overview of the Study   4
  Summary of Conclusions   9

2 BACKGROUND   11
  The Federal Food, Drug, and Cosmetic
     Act   13
  Meat, Poultry, and Fish Inspection   19
  Biotechnology   25
  Food Irradiation   29
  International Issues   31
  Food Labeling, Nutrition, and Safety   33
  Economic Studies of the Cost of Food
     Contamination and Food-borne
     Disease   34
  Conclusion   36

3 THE MARKET FOR FOOD SAFETY   37
  The Meaning of Safety   38
  The Demand for Food Safety   39
  Supply and Market Equilibrium   40
  Properties of Market Equilibrium   43
  Conclusion   54

4 PRINCIPLES AND TOOLS FOR EFFICIENT FOOD
  SAFETY REGULATION   56
  Regulatory Principles   56

Policy Tools for Food Safety Regulation 66
Efficient Food Safety Regulation 73
Conclusion 77

5 TOWARD REGULATORY REFORM   79
Where Is Regulation Warranted? 79
Consistency with Regulatory Principles 81
Recommendations for Regulatory
   Reform 88
Implications for the 1995 Farm Bill 91

REFERENCES   93

ABBREVIATIONS AND ACRONYMS   101

INDEX   103

ABOUT THE AUTHOR   109

TABLES
  2–1 Some Significant Events in the
       Regulation of Food Safety,
       1906–1992 12
  2–2 Dollar Costs Resulting from Food-
       borne Pathogens 35
  3–1 Efficiency of Equilibriums in the
       Market for Food Safety 55
  4–1 Approaches to the Control of Risk 66
  4–2 Efficient Policy Tools in the Market for
       Food Safety 78

FIGURES
  3–1 Market Equilibrium Determination of
       Safety 45
  3–2 Average Cost of Safety 50
  3–3 Distributions of Risk Attitudes or
       Vulnerabilities in the Consumer
       Population 51

Foreword

Choice and Efficiency in Food Safety Policy, by John M. Antle, is one of eight in a series devoted to agricultural policy reform published by the American Enterprise Institute. AEI has a long tradition of contributing to the effort to understand and improve agricultural policy. AEI published books of essays before the 1977, 1981, and 1985 farm bills.

Agricultural policy has increasingly become part of the general policy debate. Whether the topic is trade policy, deregulation, or budget deficits, the same forces that affect other government programs are shaping farm policy discussions. It is fitting then for the AEI Studies in Agricultural Policy to deal with these issues with the same tools and approaches applied to other economic and social topics.

Periodic farm bills (along with budget acts) remain the principal vehicles for policy changes related to agriculture, food, and other rural issues. The 1990 farm legislation expires in 1995, and in recognition of the opportunity presented by the national debate surrounding the 1995 farm bill, the American Enterprise Institute has launched a major research project. The new farm bill will allow policy makers to bring agriculture more in line with market realities. The AEI studies were intended to capitalize on that important opportunity.

The AEI project includes studies on eight related topics prepared by recognized policy experts. Each study investigates the public rationale for government's role with respect to several agricultural issues. The authors have developed evidence on the effects of recent policies and analyzed alternatives. Most research was carried out in 1994, and draft reports were discussed at a policy research workshop held in Washington, D.C., November 3–4, 1994.

The individual topics include investigation of:

- the rationale for and consequences of farm programs in general
- specific reforms of current farm programs appropriate for 1995, including analysis of individual programs for grains, milk, cotton, and sugar, among others
- agricultural trade policy for commodities in the context of recent multilateral trade agreements, with attention both to long-run goals of free trade and to intermediate steps
- crop insurance and disaster aid policy
- the government's role in conservation of natural resources and the environmental consequences of farm programs
- farm credit policy, including analysis of both subsidy and regulation
- food safety policy
- the role of public R & D policy for agriculture, what parts of the research portfolio should be subsidized, and how the payoff to publicly supported science can be improved through better policy

John Antle investigates economic principles that guide food safety policy. He asks what underlies the rationale for the role of government in food safety regulation. From this basic economic approach, he argues that food inspection policy and food regulations should be streamlined and consolidated. In addition to broad principles, the author deals with specific issues such as meat and poultry inspection to prevent disease outbreaks, food labeling to provide information to consumers, and regulations about what information firms may provide to their customers. Policy reform in food safety will likely not be accomplished easily or quickly. This study will be useful in the current debate and in the years to come.

Selected government policy may be helpful in allowing agriculture to become more efficient and effective. Unfortunately, most agricultural policy in the United States fails in that respect. In many ways, the policies of the past six decades have been counterproductive and counter to productivity. Now, in the final few years of the twentieth century, flaws in policies developed decades ago are finally becoming so obvious that farm policy observers and participants are willing to consider even eliminating many traditional subsidies and regulations. In the current context, another round of minor fixes is now seen as insufficient.

In 1995, Congress seems ready to ask tough questions about agricultural policy. How much reform is forthcoming, however, and which specific changes will be accomplished are not settled and depend on the information and analysis available to help guide the process. Understanding the consequences of alternative public policies is important. The AEI Studies in Agricultural Policy are designed to aid the process now and for the future by improving the knowledge base on which public policy is built.

CHRISTOPHER DeMUTH
American Enterprise Institute
for Public Policy Research

1
Introduction

Food safety is a goal everyone shares. But a food supply that is 100 percent safe is an unattainable goal, and improving the safety of food is costly. Choices must be made between different dimensions of food safety—for example, between the regulation of pesticide use and the prevention of food-borne illness—and also between a safer food supply and other uses of public and private resources. The more efficiently society's demand for food safety is met, the more resources are available for other uses.

The concepts of choice and efficiency, however, have not played a central role in the design of most legislation dealing with human health risk and food safety. Most legislation is written, and most regulatory decisions are taken, without explicit recognition of the choices that have to be made within the regulation domain of food safety or between food safety and other goals. These choices are therefore made implicitly, and the outcomes often yield surprising, costly, and in some cases deadly consequences.

Today heart disease and cancer are the leading causes of death in the United States; 25 percent of Americans die from some form of cancer. Experts increasingly recognize that certain types of behavior—diet, smoking, and lifestyle—are strongly associated with the risk of various types of cancer. This knowledge provides individuals with many opportunities to reduce the risk of death from cancer at relatively low cost. Put in terms of a lifetime risk of death, all forms of cancer represent a risk of 250,000 in 1 million. The Centers for Disease Control estimates that 9,000 deaths per year are associated with food-borne disease, at a risk of about 2,400 in 1 million over a seventy-year lifetime. At the same time, the Environmental Protection Agency's regulation of agricultural pesticides has attempted to achieve a lifetime cancer mortality risk of 1-in-1 million or less. Estimates based on actual pesticide residues in food indicate that fewer than 10 excess cancers per year may be caused by pesticide residues.

Clearly, unless the cost of reducing an additional death from heart disease, cancer, or food-borne disease were thousands of times higher than the cost of reducing the risk of a cancer death from pesticide residues, the current emphasis in food safety regulation on prevention of cancer from chemical residues represents a wildly inefficient allocation of public funds. This inefficiency exists within the food safety domain, as well as between that area and other areas of health and safety policy. Such misregulation is more than an academic or even an economic issue—it is undoubtedly costing American lives every year. Ironically, pesticide regulations themselves raise the cost of one method of averting heart disease and cancer—consuming a diet rich in fruits and vegetables—and thus discourage behavior that lowers the risk of these diseases.

How can this seemingly absurd situation result from well-meaning food safety legislation? One answer is that federal legislation does not require an efficient allocation of resources among the various aspects of food safety and health policy. Only coincidentally are health and safety regulations efficient in the sense that the last dollar spent on each program yields the same risk reduction. In addition, most food safety regulation is based on a paternalistic view of government—the view that government can make food safety choices better for people than they can make for themselves. This paternalism then becomes an excuse for inefficiency—people cannot choose for themselves, so it is better to have inefficient government regulations protecting people than to leave them at the mercy of the marketplace.

An equally important but more subtle source of inefficiency is the type of regulations that are typically imposed by agencies such as the Food and Drug Administration. One of the FDA's principal regulatory tools is the imposition of good manufacturing practices, that is, prescriptions for how the production process should be designed and managed. One major lesson of the past two decades of environmental regulation is that design standards are a notoriously *inefficient* way to achieve regulatory goals. Every firm's plant, equipment, and management are different, and it is impossible for bureaucrats to tailor design standards that would be efficient for every firm. Inflexible design standards discourage innovation, the key source of long-term productivity growth. To the extent that conforming to design standards is a fixed cost independent of plant size, such standards also tend to put small firms at a competitive disadvantage relative to larger firms.

The importance of these factors is underscored by the intention of the FDA and the U.S. Department of Agriculture (USDA) to mandate the Hazard Analysis Critical Control Points (HACCP) system of quality control for the entire food industry (FDA 1994c; USDA 1995). Advocates of HACCP argue that it has been successfully used in the food industry for several decades. But HACCP advocates seem to ignore the difference between a technology voluntarily adopted by a firm and tailored to its needs and one designed and enforced by government bureaucrats and inspectors. Moreover, because compliance with HACCP regulations involves a significant start-up cost that is independent of size of operation, the economic survival of small firms may be at stake.

3

There is widespread sentiment that it is time to re-consider the design of food and agricultural policy in the United States. Partly this view is brought about by the recognition that the commodity emphasis of U.S. agricultural policy is an anachronism of Great Depression–era policies; partly it is brought about by the recognition that government regulation is often costly and ineffective. But the desire for the reform of food policy is also brought about by the changing priorities of the public. As real incomes grow both domestically and internationally, people place more emphasis on the quality of food consumed and less on the quantity.

The purpose of this study is to take a fresh look at issues of food safety policy from an economic perspective. We consider the following questions:

• What are the key issues of food safety, and how do federal policies address them?

• Under what conditions—what aspects of safety, consumer behavior and knowledge, and market conditions—is regulation of food safety needed?

• What economic principles should guide the design of food safety regulation when it is needed?

• What kinds of changes in existing legislation would move the current system toward the goal of a safer food supply at lower cost?

• What role should farm bill legislation play in achieving food safety policy goals?

Overview of the Study

Chapter 2 provides background on the legislation and issues that arise in food safety policy. Existing food safety legislation addresses a wide array of issues, including the quality and safety of whole foods and food additives; inspection of animals and fish for disease; food contamination by microbial pathogens, chemical residues, and physical hazards; the safety of new foods and food production processes, including the use of genetic engineering and irradiation; effects of diet on health; nutrition; safety labeling of foods; and the international trade implications of food safety regulations.

A complex array of laws has evolved since the early part of this century to deal with the various aspects of food safety regulation. The principal responsibility for food safety regulation lies with the Food and Drug Administration, under the authority of the Pure Food and Drugs Act of 1906 and its amendments. These activities include setting regulatory standards for the safety of whole foods and food additives, developing good management practices for food processing, food labeling, and fish and seafood inspection. The FDA must approve genetically engineered foods and food products and other new technologies such as irradiation. The U.S. Department of Agriculture's Food Safety Inspection Service and other USDA agencies, under the authority of a number of laws, conduct meat, poultry, and egg inspection, testing, and labeling programs; oversee various research and education programs; and manage testing programs for food imports. The Environmental Protection Agency is responsible for pesticide regulation under the Federal Insecticide, Fungicide, and Rodenticide Act and its amendments.

Numerous studies have estimated the total costs of food-borne diseases to be in the tens of billions of dollars annually. Some attempts have been made to estimate the benefits of reduced disease associated with improved diet, and the findings indicate that these benefits are also likely to be worth billions of dollars, although comprehensive estimates are not yet available. Estimates of the costs associated with cancers caused by pesticide residues in foods, however, are controversial, as they are based on a number of assumptions to predict cancers. Estimates based on EPA methods are about 1,000 times higher than the estimates based on actual food residues.

5

The food residue methods imply that pesticide residues in foods cause about six excess cancers per year in the United States.

Chapter 3 provides an economic analysis of the market for food safety. With perfect (or sufficiently good) information about product quality, the interplay of demand and supply for food products results in an efficient provision of safety—the amount of safety consumers are both willing and able to pay for. But food product markets can efficiently provide food safety under other common conditions. When products are purchased repeatedly or low-cost product information is available, and when consumers can ascertain product quality either before or after purchase, firms can establish reputations for product quality and can charge a higher price for high-quality products. In addition, markets can function efficiently when a sufficient number of knowledgeable consumers exist to generate a demand for safety that is representative of the preferences of the general population.

The analysis in chapter 3 also finds that food product markets may be inefficient under several circumstances: when information is imperfect, consumers purchase a product only once, and information costs are high; when information is imperfect for consumers both before and after purchase; and when a majority of consumers are unknowledgeable about product safety attributes.

Considering that a relatively large proportion of the population is knowledgeable about food safety and that many food purchases are repeat purchases or relatively low-cost information is available, economic theory predicts that the unregulated market is likely to meet the food safety demands of the public efficiently. The one place where the market is likely to fail is where there is imperfect information before and after purchase. This case of imperfect pre- and postmarket information is an important one, however, as it represents the situation with many food-borne diseases and the effects of chronic exposure, such as cancer, that may be caused by chemical contamination.

Chapter 4 begins with a discussion of economic principles that should guide the design of food safety regulations: regulations must pass a benefit-cost analysis test that should be conducted independently of regulatory agencies; uncertainty associated with estimation of both benefits and costs of regulation must be treated consistently in regulatory benefit-cost analysis; individual choice is generally more efficient than uniform statutory risk standards; and incentive-based regulation is generally more efficient than command-and-control, design-standard regulation.

These principles are used to identify the efficient forms of regulation to counteract an inefficient solution of an unregulated market. For most cases, education, labeling, and liability are efficient solutions. Even when consumers have imperfect information before and after the purchase of a product, as long as producers and sellers have quality information, product-labeling requirements can solve the consumer's information problem. The one class of problems where statutory regulation is indicated as possibly being the efficient solution is when *both* consumers and producers have imperfect information about product quality. In that case, firms cannot reveal quality information under a labeling law because they do not have it.

Chapter 5 assesses the current regulatory system. Where is regulation warranted? The answer, provided by the analyses of chapters 3 and 4, is only when labeling and education cannot provide the information and knowledge that consumers need to make wise food safety choices. Food-borne diseases and chemical contamination fall into this category. The analysis of efficient regulatory principles and tools suggests, therefore, that performance standards should be used when they can pass a benefit-cost analysis test.

Chapter 5 discusses the consistency of existing laws and regulations with the principles outlined in chapter 4. Existing executive orders require that regulations are subjected to benefit-cost analyses, but because these analyses are conducted by the regulatory agency itself, they are likely to be biased in favor of regulation. Some aspects of pesticide regulation allow the benefits of regulations to be balanced against costs, although the health effects of pesticides are inflated with arbitrary uncertainty factors, while costs of restricting the use of the pesticides are not. Again, the system is biased in favor of regulation.

Existing nutrition-labeling policy, the USDA's recent meat-labeling regulations, and the various consumer education programs are broadly consistent with the principles and analyses of this study. Most statutory food safety regulations under the Federal Food, Drug, and Cosmetic Act of 1938 (FFDCA), however, are broadly inconsistent with the conclusions of the analysis of chapters 3 and 4. The FDA requires food-processing plants to conform to good management practices, a type of design standard. The FDA is now developing HACCP regulations for fish and seafood and plans to impose HACCP regulations on the entire food industry. These regulations are likely to take the form of design standards, and the choice of hazards to be controlled will not be subjected to independent benefit-cost analyses. Thus, these HACCP regulations are likely to be broadly *inconsistent* with the principles of efficient regulation outlined in chapter 4. In addition, the Delaney clause of the FFDCA remains the outstanding example of inefficient regulation in the food safety area, with its requirement that pesticides meet a "conservatively" estimated zero-risk standard for cancer.

Summary of Conclusions

Efficient regulation of food safety is a desirable social goal because it means that more safety is obtained—there are fewer illnesses and deaths from food risks—at every level of regulatory effort. A truly efficient system of food safety regulation would also select the level of regulatory effort that gives people the opportunity to obtain the degree of safety that they are willing and able to pay for.

Inefficient regulation means that consumers are not obtaining the degree of safety that they are willing to pay for and that what safety they are obtaining is costing them more than necessary. This study finds that the current food safety system in the United States is inefficient for a variety of reasons, the principal ones being

- a misallocation of effort: too much effort devoted to avoidance of cancer risk from chemical residues, too little effort devoted to risks associated with food-borne diseases and diseases associated with diet
- an overreliance on statutory regulation in general and on outmoded and inefficient process design standards in particular
- an underreliance on incentives for firms and informed individual choice for consumers (education and product labeling)

Yet the elements of a more efficient system are in place, a system that could produce the degree of safety that consumers are willing and able to pay for at minimum cost to both consumers and producers. Based on the background and analyses presented in this study, chapter 5 presents a series of recommendations for the reform of food safety policy. These recommendations, in summary form, follow:

- Conduct an independent assessment of priorities to achieve an efficient use of resources across major areas

9

of concern—dietary causes of disease, biological hazards and food-borne disease, and chemical contamination— and amend existing legislation to allow regulatory agencies to allocate effort accordingly.

• Make the first priority of food safety policy to expand research and education to enhance the capacity of producers and consumers to make informed safety choices.

• Replace outdated and inefficient design standards with a combination of safety labeling and efficient performance standards that pass an objective benefit-cost test. In particular, subject proposed HACCP regulations to independent benefit-cost analysis tests.

Food safety policy has not traditionally been a major part of farm legislation. Clearly, this study's recommendation that research, consumer education, and labeling substitute for statutory regulation is consistent with the research and education titles of past farm bills. Many who argue for the consolidation of responsibility of food safety regulation in one agency, however, do not necessarily advocate that these responsibilities be assigned to the USDA. But unless this single-agency model becomes a reality, there does appear to be the opportunity to use the farm bill as a vehicle for reform of at least those parts of the food safety regulatory system—notably, meat and poultry inspection—for which the USDA currently has responsibility.

The simple message of this study is that we can have safer food at lower cost, by simply putting basic economic considerations into the priority setting, design, and implementation of food safety policy.

2
Background

The modern era of food safety regulation in the United States began with the passage of the Pure Food and Drugs Act of 1906 and the Meat Inspection Act of 1906. Periodic amendments to these acts occurred in 1938, in the 1950s, and subsequently. Other major laws are the Federal Insecticide, Fungicide, and Rodenticide Act of 1947 (FIFRA) and its amendments and the Wholesome Meat Act of 1967. For a history of the Meat Inspection Act, see Libecap (1992). Middlekauff (1989) provides a review of these laws and their amendments, summarized in table 2–1.

The Federal Food, Drug, and Cosmetic Act (FFDCA) gives the major responsibility for general food safety, as well as seafood safety and inspection, to the Food and Drug Administration. The Commerce Department's National Marine Fisheries Service conducts fish products inspection and grading. Meat, poultry, and egg inspection and related research and education are the responsibility of the U.S. Department of Agriculture's Food Safety Inspection Service (FSIS). The USDA's Animal and Plant Health Inspection Service has responsibility for programs related to plant health, plant pests and diseases, pest management, and animal disease control, including testing and quarantine of imports. The Environmental Protection Agency is responsible for pesticide regulation, in the areas of human health and the environment, under FIFRA and section 408 of FFDCA. The U.S. Department of Treasury's Bureau of Alcohol, Tobacco, and Firearms

TABLE 2–1

SOME SIGNIFICANT EVENTS IN THE REGULATION OF FOOD SAFETY,
1906–1992

Year	Event	Year	Event
1906	Pure Food and Drugs Act of 1906 and Meat Inspection Act of 1906 enacted.	1968	Wholesome Poultry Products Act enacted.
1927	Food, Drug, and Insecticide Administration (renamed Food and Drug Administration in 1931) became a separate unit of the U.S. Department of Agriculture.	1969	Good manufacturing practices regulations first adopted.
		1970	Egg Products Inspection Act enacted.
1938	Federal Food, Drug, and Cosmetic Act of 1938 enacted.	1975	Corporate officer criminally convicted for sanitation problem in food-containing facility.
1946	Agricultural Marketing Act enacted.	1985	FDA proposes *de minimis* exception to Delaney clause for a food additive in its entirety to allow continued use of methylene chloride to decaffeinate coffee.
1947	Federal Insecticide, Fungicide, and Rodenticide Act enacted.		
1953	Congress gave FDA authority to inspect a plant, after written notice to the owner, without a warrant and without permission of the owner.	1986	FDA stated that food produced by new biotechnology could result in a level of substance that "may be injurious to health."
1957	Poultry Products Inspection Act enacted.	1990	Nutrition Labeling and Education Act enacted.
1958	Food Additives Amendment of 1958 enacted.	1992	U.S. Ninth Circuit Court of Appeals overturned EPA's use of *de minimis* standard for pesticide cancer risk.
1967	Wholesome Meat Act enacted.		

SOURCE: Middlekauff (1989).

is responsible for ingredients in alcoholic beverages and tobacco products.

The FDA and the USDA also are responsible for food labeling. The FSIS is responsible for regulation of meat and poultry product labels pursuant to the Federal Meat Inspection Act and the Poultry Products Inspection Act. Under FFDCA, the FDA has responsibility for most other food labeling. The Nutrition Labeling and Education Act of 1990 directed the FDA to improve nutrition labels, a task completed in May 1984.

The Federal Food, Drug, and Cosmetic Act

The original 1906 act aimed to protect the public by prohibiting the sale of adulterated food, that is, food that contained "any added poisonous or other added deleterious ingredient which may render such article injurious to health." The ambiguity of this concept led to subsequent laws that strengthened and clarified food safety concepts.

For example, the 1938 act states that a food is adulterated if it is a "filthy, putrid, or decomposed substance, or if it is otherwise unfit." Moreover, any food prepared, packed, or held under insanitary conditions, whether or not any contamination occurs, is also considered adulterated. Accordingly, the FDA has promulgated good manufacturing practice regulations. These regulations specify aspects of the manufacturing process, such as requirements for cleanliness, design of equipment, maintenance, and development of quality control procedures. The 1938 act also outlaws economic adulteration, that is, adding something to food to make it appear to have greater value than it does.

A major revision of the law took place in 1958, when the food additives amendment established the requirement of safety. Whereas the FDA had been required to prove adulteration with an emphasis on the quality of whole food (section 402), the new law required that industry prove the safety of additives (section 409). Safety was defined as "reasonable certainty that no harm will result from the proposed use of an additive." This requirement was generally interpreted to mean that a safe additive was associated with a zero degree of risk (Middlekauff 1989).

To prevent the food additives amendment from requiring that all food ingredients in use in 1958 be evaluated as additives, ingredients that had received prior sanction were exempted from section 409. In addition, substances that were considered "generally recognized as safe," based on common use or scientific data, were exempted from section 409.

Pesticide Regulation and the Delaney Clause. All pesticides registered for use on food crops in the United States must be granted a tolerance by the Environmental Protection Agency. Tolerances are the most important tool the U.S. government has to regulate pesticide residues in food (National Research Council 1993). Tolerances, the maximum quantity of a pesticide residue allowable, are set both for raw commodities under section 408 of FFDCA and for processed foods in which pesticides concentrate under section 409. Tolerances are proposed by manufacturers of pesticides based on good agricultural practices for each use of a pesticide. Thus, if a pesticide is used on five different crops, five tolerances must be approved.

Toxicological studies of animals, and when possible humans, are used to determine safe levels of residue exposure, for both acute and chronic effects. These studies are used to set a *reference dose* against which expected exposure can be compared. The reference dose is calculated as the no-observed-adverse-effect-level (the highest dose at which there is no statistically significant adverse effect in test animals beyond that exhibited in a control

14

group), adjusted by an uncertainty factor associated with the extrapolation of experimental animal data to humans. The reference dose is compared with expected exposure, based on food consumption and food residues. When anticipated exposure exceeds the reference dose, the proposed tolerance is rejected, and the manufacturer seeking registration may recommend a new tolerance.

The 1958 amendments to FFDCA give the EPA the authority to set tolerances, or maximum allowable levels, for pesticide residues in foods. Section 408 concerns tolerances for residues in or on raw commodities and allows risks to be balanced against potential benefits of the pesticide. Section 409 applies to pesticide residues in processed foods and treats them as food additives. Section 409 also contains the Delaney clause, which provides "that no additive shall be deemed to be safe if it is found to induce cancer when ingested by man or animal, or if it is found, after tests which are appropriate for the evaluation of the safety of food additives, to induce cancer in man or animals." Consequently, section 409 has been interpreted as applying a zero-risk standard for pesticides that concentrate in processed foods, without provision for cancer risks to be balanced against potential benefits of the pesticide.

When the Delaney clause was written into law, analysts could detect quantities of impurities in microgram amounts (one part per million). By the 1970s, because of the introduction of high-performance liquid chromatography, the detection limits had decreased to nanograms (parts per billion). A combination of gas chromatography and mass spectrometry lowered the limit to picograms (parts per trillion, or 10^{-12}). Limits can now be pushed to 10^{-15}, 10^{-18}, and even 10^{-21}, which is near the molecular level (Francis 1992). Thus, since the 1950s, when it was meaningful to ask whether or not a compound was present, the relevant scientific and risk-assessment question has become whether or not a compound can be used

15

safely. Unfortunately, FFDCA remains based on the concepts of the 1950s.

Until the mid-1980s, the EPA used a strict zero-risk interpretation of the Delaney clause. Consequently, it did not register new pesticides if the chemical was considered a potential carcinogen. Yet the EPA was not revoking registration of pesticides that were previously registered and had section 409 tolerances established, even if tests had subsequently shown the pesticide to be a potential carcinogen. Often newer pesticides that were denied registration exhibited much lower cancer risk than the older ones. But because the Delaney clause does not allow balancing benefits and costs, the newer lower-risk materials could not be substituted for the older ones.

In its 1987 report, the National Research Council recommended that the Delaney clause be replaced with a negligible-risk standard for both raw and processed foods. The NRC report observed that 55 percent of total dietary cancer risk for the twenty-eight pesticides studied would be eliminated by strict application of the Delaney clause. Yet the NRC study found that a 98 percent reduction in cancer risk would be attained from adoption of a uniform negligible-risk standard applied to both raw and processed foods. The conclusions of the NRC study were subsequently criticized for excessively pessimistic exposure assumptions, which themselves overstate true dietary cancer risk (Archibald and Winter 1990). Nevertheless, it should still be true that a negligible-risk standard, though possibly unnecessarily strict as interpreted by the EPA, would be a significant improvement over the stringent application of the Delaney clause.

The EPA subsequently announced in October 1988 that it would provide a *de minimis* exemption to the Delaney clause, that is, an exemption based on the case law premise that an agency need not apply a statute literally when it yields pointless results. The EPA defined a negligible or *de minimis* risk as one cancer per million persons exposed to a pesticide through food consumption during a seventy-year lifetime. Importantly, even this *de minimis* standard is conservative, as it is based on a variety of worst-case assumptions. Thus, the 1-in-1 million lifetime risk is an upper bound of potential cancer risk, with the true risk likely to be much lower and in some cases zero. As an indication of how conservative the *de minimis* standard is, the general risk of cancer in the United States population is about 25 percent, or 250,000 per million.

In July 1992 the U.S. Ninth Circuit Court of Appeals ruled on a petition filed by several organizations and individuals asking the EPA to revoke the tolerances for seven potentially carcinogenic pesticides on the basis of the Delaney clause. The court ruling overturned the EPA's use of its *de minimis* standard for cancer risk for four of the seven pesticides in the petition. This ruling opened the possibility that more than thirty other pesticides' section 409 tolerances, as well as section 408 tolerances, could be revoked, according to the EPA (Winter 1993).

In 1990 the Bush administration proposed to amend FFDCA by adopting the National Research Council's recommendation that a negligible risk standard replace the Delaney clause. Moreover, the administration proposed to apply, when a risk is found to be greater than negligible, the same balancing of health benefits against regulatory costs that is applied in regulation of residues in raw agricultural commodities. Congress did not act on these recommendations.

In 1994 the Clinton administration proposed a negligible-risk standard to replace the Delaney clause in FFDCA as well as the setting of tolerances for raw agricultural commodities. The new standard would require "a reasonable certainty of no harm," and the interpretation of this in numerical terms is not specified. Thus, the Clinton proposal would eliminate the consideration of pesticide benefits from all pesticide tolerance-setting decisions. The standard would consider health risks only. ✓ The Clinton proposal also adopts some NRC recommendations that differences in exposure between children and adults be taken into consideration in setting tolerances (Kuchler et al. 1994). The likely result of this change would be to tighten further the standards for pesticide registration.

The Federal Insecticide, Fungicide, and Rodenticide Act. FIFRA, with its comprehensive amendments of 1972, 1975, 1978, 1980, and 1988, is the principal federal legislation regulating pesticides, in addition to sections 408 and 409 of FFDCA. The 1972 amendments made FIFRA a unique piece of environmental and safety legislation: they required pesticides to be regulated to avoid "unacceptable adverse effects on the environment," defined as "any unreasonable risk to man or the environment, taking into account the economic, social, and environmental costs and benefits of any pesticide." According to the study by Cropper and others (1992), in practice pesticide registration decisions have indeed reflected, at least to a degree, the potential benefits and costs of the pesticides that were considered for registration.

The 1972 amendments also provided for a pesticide registration process for all pesticides in use in the United States. A pesticide must be registered for each use, that is, for each crop to which it may be applied. General registration requires labeling with approved uses and safety precautions; restricted registration, for more hazardous materials, allows use only by certified applicators. The 1972 amendment required that the approximately 40,000 products on the market be reregistered, but the EPA could not complete this process. The 1978 amendments to FIFRA simplified the task by focusing reregistration on the approximately 600 active ingredients used in pes-

18

ticides. In 1984, registration standards were updated to reflect new environmental and health data.

The 1988 amendments to FIFRA directed that by 1997 the EPA should reregister all pesticides registered before 1984. Registrants were required to provide all environmental and health data required for new pesticides and to pay for costs of reregistration. Yet as of the end of 1993, only 17 of the 194 pesticides considered high-priority had undergone initial reviews. One reason for the slow progress in completing reregistration is the cost and complexity of the risk-benefit trade-offs that must be assessed by the EPA (Kuchler et al. 1994).

One of the problems created by the lengthy and costly reregistration process is the loss of reregistrations for "minor use" pesticides. Manufacturers often cannot afford to reregister pesticides that are not used in large quantities. The producers of these minor-use crops—primarily certain vegetables, fruits, and ornamentals—thus risk losing pesticides that are valuable tools for pest control and in some cases have no close substitutes (Council for Agricultural Science and Technology 1992).

In 1990 the Bush administration proposed to simplify pesticide registration procedures and to establish a periodic review of all pesticides. Similarly, the Clinton administration has proposed establishing a periodic review (every fifteen years) of all pesticides and a priority process for reduced-risk and minor-use pesticides. The proposal would also allow the EPA to give conditional registrations before completion of tests for biologically based pesticides.

Meat, Poultry, and Fish Inspection

Modern meat inspection law began with the Federal Meat Inspection Act of 1906. The act required inspection of all meat intended for interstate and foreign commerce, including antemortem inspection, postmortem inspection, and inspection at all stages of processing and inspection of meat-packing equipment and facilities. Current law is governed by the various amendments to the 1906 act, notably the Wholesome Meat Act of 1967 and the Wholesome Poultry Products Act of 1986, which extended meat inspection to products in intrastate commerce and included all meat and poultry.

These statutes require the Food Safety and Inspection Service of the USDA (and the Agricultural Marketing Service in the case of eggs and egg products) to inspect slaughterhouses, meat and poultry processing plants, and egg packing and processing plants. Inspection of slaughtering plants is continuous, and a federal inspector must be present at all times. The FSIS employs more than 8,000 inspectors and veterinary medical officers. Food processing plants are inspected by some 900 FDA inspectors (Gantz 1990).

FSIS inspection is based primarily on organoleptic surveillance methods (that is, sight, smell, and touch). While this approach made sense at the turn of the century when few other methods were available, it is widely recognized by the scientific community that these inspections are incapable of detecting disease-causing microorganisms or chemical contamination. Moreover, critics have cited the inability of the meat inspection system to keep up with processing technology advances such as higher-speed equipment and with new risks from contamination by pesticides, drugs, and environmental contaminants.

Although the meat inspection system has been subjected to periodic criticism for many years, this criticism reached a head in early 1993, when some 500 people in the northwestern United States contracted *E. coli* from contaminated ground beef and three children and one adult died. In response to the public attention to these poisonings, the USDA announced the development of a rapid (five-minute) test for microbial contamination. In

September 1994 Secretary of Agriculture Michael Espy announced that the Clinton administration was proposing a Pathogen Reduction Act to require microbial testing in meat and poultry inspection.

The Application of HACCP in Inspection Programs. The National Research Council's (1985) study of FSIS's meat inspection programs and poultry inspection (NRC 1987) recommended that the FSIS adopt the Hazard Analysis Critical Control Points, or HACCP, system to modernize its inspection programs. HACCP was developed by Pillsbury in the 1960s to ensure quality in the production of food for the space program. According to the draft HACCP principles of the Codex Committee on Food Hygiene (Pierson and Corlett 1992):

> HACCP is a system which identifies specific hazard(s) (i.e., any biological, chemical, or physical property that adversely affects the safety of the food) and preventative measures for their control. The system consists of the following seven principles:
>
> **Principle 1**
> Identify the potential hazard(s) associated with food production at all stages, from growth, processing, manufacture and distribution, until the point of consumption. Assess the likelihood of occurrence of the hazard(s) and identify the preventative measures for their control.
>
> **Principle 2**
> Determine the points/procedures/operational steps that can be controlled to eliminate the hazard(s) or minimize its likelihood of occurrence—(Critical Control Point (CCP)). A "step" means any stage in food production and/or manufacture including raw materials, their receipt and/or production, harvesting, transport, formulation, processing, storage, etc.

21

Principle 3
Establish target level(s) and tolerances which must be met to ensure the CCP is under control.

Principle 4
Establish a monitoring system to ensure control of the CCP by scheduled testing or observations.

Principle 5
Establish the corrective action to be taken when monitoring indicates that a particular CCP is not under control.

Principle 6
Establish procedures for verification which includes supplementary tests and procedures to confirm that HACCP is working effectively.

Principle 7
Establish documentation concerning all procedures and records appropriate to these principles and their application.

Until recently, the only mandated HACCP program for food safety was for the low-acid canned food industry. The FDA imposed the system in the early 1970s in response to concerns about the contamination of canned foods with the deadly *C. botulinum* microorganism. After the NRC reports recommended the use of HACCP in meat and poultry inspection, in 1989 the FSIS embarked on a program with industry to test HACCP in volunteer plants.

There have been many unsuccessful attempts over the past two decades to pass laws reforming the way that fish and seafood safety is regulated. In January 1994 the FDA issued regulations for a mandatory HACCP program for fish and seafood inspection under the authority of FFDCA (FDA 1994b). The final regulations are expected to be announced by the FDA in 1995. In August 1994 the FDA's commissioner, David Kessler, announced that the FDA planned to extend HACCP to all food production, including meat and poultry inspection, although it was unclear where the FDA thought its authority ended and the USDA's began. These proposed regulations were announced in August 1994 FDA 1994c).

HACCP implementation in meat, poultry, and seafood inspection raises a number of important questions. First, the scientific basis of HACCP is the hazard analysis or risk assessment component. It is not clear that the federal agencies have the capability or the data needed to identify the most important health effects posed by the various hazards—hazards that range from microorganisms and parasites to chemical residues and naturally occurring toxins to hazards from physical contaminants such as glass particles. Experts do not know what proportion of major food-borne diseases such as *Salmonella* or *Campylobacter* are attributable to different types of meats and poultry and would not be able to determine the possible effects of HACCP on health risk in the general population. Consumer groups, such as the Safe Food Coalition, are concerned that HACCP will result in a relaxation of safety inspection standards, with industry recordkeeping replacing federal inspectors.

There is the concern in the industry that the development and monitoring of HACCP will be costly, and that it will be unable to keep up with technological advances in the food industry (Becker 1992). Another major industry concern with HACCP is that, with the exception of the low-acid canned food HACCP, HACCP has been successful only when it was voluntarily adopted by industry. When firms choose to design a HACCP system, they are free to select those control points that provide a cost-effective means of achieving their quality goals. When a HACCP system is mandated by government regulations, however, government bureaucrats must write design standards that apply to every firm in the industry, and these bureaucrats lack both the information and the incentive to ensure that the outcome is cost-effective. In its comments on the FDA's proposed mandatory HACCP regulations for fish and seafood, the president of the American Frozen Food Institute, S. C. Anderson, commented:

> AFFI members always have endorsed the voluntary assimilation of HACCP principles into frozen foods operations. In fact, a recent poll conducted by the Institute indicated over 90 percent of respondents have incorporated or are in the process of incorporating HACCP into operational plans. . . . AFFI believes HACCP programs should be implemented on a voluntary basis for the vast majority of the food industry. AFFI believes for fish and fishery products, mandatory programs should be required by the regulatory agencies only in circumstances in which fish or seafood contains a sensitive ingredient which does not undergo further processing and for which a substantial body of evidence exists, based on epidemiological, scientific, and clinical data, that the fish or seafood may present a significant risk to the public health. . . . Adoption of a voluntary/mandatory HACCP program, as stipulated above, will maximize limited resources available to both the Agency and the industry, thus coordinating efforts to focus on the most pressing seafood safety concerns. Mandatory adoption of HACCP as suggested in FDA's proposal would overwhelm the system with undertrained and inexperienced FDA and industry HACCP "experts," thereby undermining HACCP programs before they have even become effective. . . . It is unclear from the proposal that a "mandatory HACCP requirement" for low risk products such as frozen fish and seafood advances the "protection of public health." (Anderson 1994)

24

A HACCP system can also be defined as a set of performance standards for different stages in the production, processing, and marketing of food. This version of HACCP is more appropriate for regulatory purposes, as we discuss in chapter 4, and is similar to a voluntary HACCP program in that firms are allowed to design their quality control system to suit their particular production systems.

Another important aspect of the proposed HACCP regulations concerns their effect on small firms. According to the FDA's regulatory impact analysis, 80 percent of the seafood processors covered by the regulations have less than $1 million in annual gross revenue (less than $2 million for shrimp processing firms). Because monitoring and recordkeeping requirements of the regulations are largely fixed costs, the average cost per unit of production is higher for these small firms than for larger firms. Thus, the regulations are likely to have a disproportionately large economic impact on small firms.

Biotechnology

Genetic engineering involves the manipulation of genetic information by means of techniques other than the classic Mendelian breeding techniques that have been used for hundreds of years. Such engineering includes materials derived through genetic transformation and recombinant deoxyribonucleic acid (rDNA) technology. Initial genetic engineering work in plant biotechnology focused on improving agronomic traits of crops, for example, through the development of herbicide-tolerant and insect- and disease-resistant varieties, and tolerance to environmental stress, such as salinity, drought, or temperature extremes. Genetic engineering has also attempted to modify the nutritional and processing characteristics of food plants and extend their shelf life. Plants may also be useful vehicles for the manufacture of products such as food enzymes and industrial oils.

25

Traditional plant breeding primarily involves the exchange of genetic material between sexually compatible plants, usually members of the same species. But rDNA techniques allow the transfer of genetic material across sexual barriers that has been isolated from other plants and unrelated organisms (Olempska-Beer et al. 1993). Another key difference between the classic breeding methods and genetic engineering is the speed and precision with which key genes can be identified. Classical breeding, for example, might take seven or more generations, or selection cycles, to identify a plant with the desired characteristics. Genetic engineering techniques, by contrast, make it possible to introduce new genes from more sources without carrying in undesirable genes. But genetic engineering techniques might have unforeseen effects on the host plant and therefore must be analyzed by plant breeders as thoroughly as plants derived from classical methods. Besides increasing the speed and precision of producing plants with desirable traits similar to those that can be produced with classical methods, genetic engineering techniques also permit breeders to transfer novel genes into plants that cannot be developed by traditional breeding methods. Consequently, questions have been raised about the safety of foods derived from genetic engineering techniques (Barefoot, Beachy, and Lilburn 1994).

Recombinant DNA techniques are used to introduce genes for specific functional proteins and are also used to introduce antisense RNA (a gene introduced in a reverse orientation to inhibit expression of the endogenous sense gene). While RNA is a component of all foods, introducing new gene functions or inhibiting the functioning of a gene may result in unintended effects. These effects may include changes in nutrient content, an increase in the level of unsafe toxicants or metabolites, or a change in the allergenicity of the protein.

The source of the introduced protein is considered a

key safety consideration. Proteins derived from commonly consumed foods should generally be safe unless they possess adverse characteristics. Proteins derived from nonfood sources should be safe if they are structurally similar to proteins contained in foods. Because the function of many proteins is as yet unknown, the safety of these proteins requires analysis to determine whether their functions raise safety concerns (Olempska-Beer et al. 1993).

Biotechnology Regulation. The FFDCA gives the FDA the primary responsibility for assuring the safety of commercial foods and food additives. The safety of whole foods is addressed in section 402; section 409 of the 1958 Food Additives Amendment requires that producers and processors of food demonstrate the safety of additives to the FDA. The Animal and Plant Health Inspection Service of the USDA is also involved in biotechnology regulation, for example, when recombinantly derived materials are used to treat animals. The EPA may also be involved under FIFRA when genes have pesticidal properties.

According to the FDA's 1992 policy statement on foods derived from new plant varieties (FDA 1992), genetically engineered plant foods will be reviewed under current regulations for plant varieties produced by traditional breeding techniques. Under FFDCA these regulations involve the premarket review and approval of substances not generally recognized as safe that are added to food and postmarket authority to remove foods that pose a health hazard.

The FDA has also determined that new varieties developed by genetic engineering techniques are not required to be labeled as to development process. Thus genetically engineered plants receive the same treatment as plants derived from traditional breeding techniques. This policy is receiving further consideration by the FDA (Newsome 1993).

There is a clear rationale for the focus on product rather than on process in food safety regulation. The safety of a food should depend on the result of specific genetic modifications, whether they are accomplished by genetic engineering techniques, classical breeding, or other techniques, and not on the process of achieving those modifications.

The BST Controversy. In addition to the application of biotechnology to the development of new plant varieties, genetic engineering techniques are being used to develop products such as drugs and growth-enhancing hormones and transgenic animal species. The first major animal development, and one that has been widely publicized and debated, is the use of recombinantly derived bovine somatotropin (rBST) to enhance dairy cow productivity (see Hallberg 1992 for a review of this issue).

Under FFDCA, the FDA requires manufacturers to demonstrate that new drugs are effective and safe for both humans and animals. The FDA granted preliminary approval of rBST for experimental use in 1986 and judged the treated cows' milk as safe. A comprehensive study of the human safety of rBST was published in 1990 (Juskevich and Guyer 1990). The conclusion from exhaustive study by the FDA was that rBST was safe whether found in milk or meat. This conclusion follows from the presence of naturally occurring BST in food and from the fact that BST is biologically inactive in humans. Nevertheless, certain individuals and groups have questioned the human safety of using rBST and have called for long-term studies of its effects before it receives approval. It has also been objected to on social and economic grounds, based on the argument that small farms and rural economies would be adversely affected, and also because the existing dairy price support mechanism would cause even larger government subsidies than at present (Douthit 1991).

Monsanto's rBST was finally approved by the FDA in 1993, but its sale was delayed by a ninety-day moratorium imposed by a provision attached to the 1993 federal budget by Representative Feingold of Wisconsin. Monsanto reported that rBST was being used by 10,000 farms on about 8 percent of dairy cows in the United States as of September 1994.

The labeling of milk produced with cows treated with rBST has also been advocated by some consumer groups but has been rejected by the FDA. As an alternative, many producers and distributors have proposed that milk produced with cows not treated with rBST be labeled as "BST Free." In February 1994 the FDA issued interim guidelines in the *Federal Register* for such labeling. These guidelines indicate that milk may not be labeled as "BGH Free," "BST Free," "rBGH Free," or "rBST Free." Milk may have a statement, however, on the label saying "from cows not treated with rBST" and "no significant difference has been shown between milk derived from rBST-treated and non-rBST treated cows." Some states have allowed such labeling, with affidavits and records verifying the nonuse of rBST, whereas other states have disallowed this labeling on the basis that it would be misleading to consumers. Monsanto has opposed any labeling and argued that it would give consumers the impression that milk produced with the use of rBST is inferior to milk not produced with it, contrary to the existing scientific evidence.

Food Irradiation

Chemical fumigation is an important method of reducing postharvest losses, ensuring hygienic quality, and facilitating trade in food and food ingredients. One of the major fumigants, ethylene dibromide (EDB) was banned from this use by the EPA in 1984. Methyl bromide, one of the other major fumigants, is scheduled to be banned in the year 2000 in the United States according to the Clean Air Act and in most European countries because it is considered to contribute to the depletion of the ozone layer. Methyl bromide is used extensively for fumigation of fruit and vegetable imports into the United States and is the only import quarantine treatment approved by the USDA. Ethylene oxide, another widely used fumigant, was banned in the European Community in 1991 and may also be banned in other countries. Thus, in the near future there may be few if any effective fumigants available for use in commercial food production.

Low-dose irradiation of food is considered an effective substitute for these broad-spectrum fumigants, and its use has been endorsed by many national and international organizations. In 1980 an expert committee of the Food and Agriculture Organization, the International Atomic Energy Commission, and the World Health Organization concluded that low-level doses of irradiation did not represent a hazard. The Codex Alimentarius Commission of the FAO/WHO Food Standard Program adopted standards for food irradiation in 1983. Thirty-seven countries have approved forty types of food for irradiation (Loaharanu 1994b).

There is general agreement among scientific groups that irradiation could yield substantial public health benefits in excess of the costs of using irradiation (Loaharanu 1994a). A study by Roberts (1985) found that the public net benefits from the use of irradiation for control of pathogens in raw meats and poultry could be $1 billion or more. Forsythe and Evangelou (1994) estimate that if methyl bromide were banned in the United States, irradiation of imported fruits and vegetables would yield net benefits of $650 million to $1.1 billion over a five-year period.

In the United States, food irradiation continues to be controversial, with certain individuals and groups opposing its use. In 1984 the FDA approved irradiation for use on food, but applications have been limited, apparently because of organized opposition to its use. In 1992 the first commercial food irradiator went into operation after considerable public debate. Irradiated fruits, vegetables, and poultry are being marketed, on a small scale, in Florida and Illinois. The recent outbreaks of foodborne disease and heightened concerns about the adequacy of inspection programs and technologies to control microbial pathogens have increased interest in the use of irradiation. The Animal and Plant Health Inspection Service, responsible for the inspection and quarantine of imported fresh fruits and vegetables, does not yet allow irradiation to be used.

International Issues

Several aspects of food safety regulation have implications for international trade in food products. The principal theme connecting all these issues is that each country has its own laws and standards regarding food quality and safety. Just as individual state standards create barriers to interstate commerce in the United States, these varying international standards complicate international trade. This issue is particularly important to international trade because quality standards can be used not only for legitimate health and safety regulation but also as nontariff barriers to restrict trade and international competition.

The Codex Alimentarius Commission was founded in 1962 by a joint commission of the FAO and WHO to provide a forum for the resolution of trade disputes that arise because of food industry regulation. Codex pursues the application of the principle of national treatment and the harmonization of minimum standards across countries, allowing countries to adopt higher standards if they so choose. Codex has standards for commodity quality, food additives, pesticide residues, and processes (primarily sanitation standards for slaughter and processing of animal products) (Skully 1994).

The United States has proposed that science-based standards be the basis of the definition of international standards for safety. This approach has been followed in the development of rules governing agricultural trade in the Uruguay Round of the General Agreement on Tariffs and Trade and in the North American Free Trade Agreement. The harmonization of health and safety standards through international trade agreements, however, is a controversial issue. Despite the principle of national treatment that allows countries to set their own standards as long as they apply the same standards to traded goods, environmental and consumer groups argue that harmonization according to Codex standards would lead to a lowering of U.S. standards.

The problem of ensuring the safety and quality of foods imported into the United States has also been controversial. The presence of chemical residues in imported foods, particularly pesticide residues in fresh fruits and vegetables, has been the subject of much public debate. The problem has come to be known as the circle of poison: U.S. firms export chemicals not approved for use in the United States, and these chemicals return to the United States as residues on imported fruits and vegetables. Legislation has been proposed to ban the export of pesticides not approved for use in the United States. The Bush administration opposed this type of legislation in 1991 on the grounds that unilateral action by the United States would not eliminate the problem but would harm the U.S. pesticide industry. Moreover, the USDA and the FDA do test imported foods for residues. Improving this testing program and strengthening penalties for violations is arguably a better solution to the problem than regulating pesticide exports (Fisher and Haley 1991). Although this type of legislation has been supported by a

32

number of consumer and environmental groups, it has not become law.

Food Labeling, Nutrition, and Safety

A number of federal regulations relate to the labeling of foods. The Fair Packaging and Labeling Act of 1966 requires that labeling information be provided to consumers in standard formats. The FDA generally disallows labels that are considered to be false or misleading; the Federal Trade Commission imposes similar standards for food advertising. Prior to 1984, FDA policy also largely prohibited health claims on labels, but the FDA issued a statement in 1987 allowing health claims on labels that follow FDA guidelines. In 1990 a new set of FDA regulations limited the types of health claims that could be made. The Nutrition Labeling and Education Act of 1990 overhauled food label law and further tightened the regulation of health claims allowed on labels; new regulations were announced in May 1994. The USDA implemented new safety labeling requirements for raw and partially cooked meat and poultry in 1994 as well.

Traditionally, food labeling has been oriented toward the provision of consumer information. The update of food labeling regulations completed in 1994 was driven by the growing evidence that major diseases, notably heart disease and cancer, are diet-related (NRC 1989). But increasingly, food labeling is regarded as a way to convey information regarding all relevant quality attributes, including safety (Caswell and Padberg 1992).

The issue of labeling also arises in the regulation of new food production and processing technologies. The labeling of genetically engineered foods and foods produced with biogenetic drugs is part of the public debate of biotechnology, as is the labeling of irradiated products. Such labeling raises a variety of issues, including

33

the provision of scientifically accurate information to consumers, industry concern that labeling will create a consumer perception biased against certain processes or products, and the costs associated with determining whether components of products are produced with a particular bioengineered product.

Economic Studies of the Cost of Food Contamination and Food-borne Disease

A number of studies have estimated costs of food-borne illness associated with the principal food-borne pathogens. A series of studies by the Economic Research Service (Roberts 1985, 1989; USDA 1993) show that the major microbial diseases cause an estimated 6.5–33 million human illnesses and 6,000 deaths. The dollar costs resulting from food-borne pathogens are estimated in the billions of dollars (table 2–2). These figures are probably underestimates because not all costs are accounted for and many cases of disease are never diagnosed or reported. According to one study that attempted to correct for underreporting, the medical costs and lost productivity costs of diarrheal disease in the United States in 1985 was on the order of $23 billion. These estimates do not count deaths, pain and suffering, liability losses, product recall, and so forth (Kvenberg and Archer 1987). Moreover, the incidence of food-borne disease is believed to be increasing in recent decades in the United States and other industrialized countries.

There is a consensus among health experts that improved diets—for example, diets with less fat and sodium and with more complex carbohydrates and fiber—would yield significant reductions in heart disease and cancer (U.S. Department of Health and Human Services 1988; NRC 1989). Comprehensive estimates of the dollar value of such benefits are not available. In its regulatory impact analysis of the seafood HACCP regula-

TABLE 2–2

DOLLAR COSTS RESULTING FROM FOOD-BORNE PATHOGENS

Pathogen	Cases	Deaths	Annual Medical and Productivity Costs ($ million)
Bacterium			
Salmonella	1,920,000	960–1,920	1,188–1,588
Campylobacter			
jejuni or coli	2,100,000	120–360	907–1,016
Escherichia coli			
0157:H7	7,668–20,448	146–389	229–610
Listeria			
monocytogenes	1,526–1,581	378–433	209–233
Parasite			
Toxoplasma gondii	2,090	42	2,628
Trichinell spiralis	131	0	0
Taenia saginata	894	0	0
Taenia solium	210	0	0

SOURCE: U.S. Department of Agriculture (1993).

tions, however, the FDA estimated that increasing fish consumption by one pound per capita per year and reducing red meat consumption by that amount, and thus reducing fat intake, would generate benefits worth more than $3 billion over a ten-year period (FDA 1994a). These estimates suggest that a more general improvement in diet could yield benefits worth billions of dollars per year.

Estimates of cancer deaths caused by chemical residues is highly controversial. According to the 1987 NRC study, which used EPA's conservative assumptions about exposure, a group of possibly carcinogenic pesticides was estimated to result in 1,462 excess deaths per year per million lifetimes. In contrast, the study by Archibald and Winter (1990), which used FDA data on actual residues in foods, estimated about 1.3 excess cancer deaths per million lifetimes for the same set of pesticides—or an estimate that differed from the NRC study by a factor of about 1,000. In 1987 the EPA estimated, according to their methods, that pesticide residues in foods caused not more than 6,000 excess cancer cases per year. Applying the factor of 1,000 derived from the Archibald and Winter analysis based on FDA residue data would yield an estimate in the range of 6. Considering that studies of the value of a statistical life give estimates on the order of $2 million (Cropper and Freeman 1991), the implied cost of pesticide cancer deaths would be $12 billion according to EPA estimates but only $12 million according to the Archibald and Winter analysis. Clearly, the "conservative" assumptions used by EPA risk-assessment procedures result in radically different estimates of cancer deaths and associated costs than do the use of actual residue data.

Conclusion

A complex array of laws and public agencies are involved in food safety regulation in the United States. These laws and institutions evolved from concerns in the early part of the century with ensuring that only healthy animals entered the food system and that processed food was not adulterated. Today, the breadth and complexity of issues have greatly expanded. Laws and regulations deal with microbial contamination of fresh and processed foods and transmission of food-borne diseases, chemical contamination of fresh and processed foods, health implications of genetically engineered foods and drugs, use of irradiation, health implications of nutrition and food labeling, and international trade issues associated with food safety regulation. Estimates of the costs of food-borne illness are on the order of billions of dollars per year. But estimates of cancer deaths associated with pesticide residues range widely, depending on whether EPA's "conservative" estimates are used or estimates are based on actual food residues.

3
The Market for Food Safety

One can buy many food products with differing safety attributes. Raw seafood is much more likely to contain food-borne disease than a well-done piece of ground beef. It is in this sense that markets exist for food safety or, more precisely, markets exist for foods with varying safety attributes. In safety as in many other aspects of life, people have differing needs and wants; business firms discern these demands in the marketplace and profit by meeting these demands.

Many choices in safety, however, are not available. Consumers will not buy a product that they consider to be unsafe. No one willingly buys contaminated meat that will cause illness or death; firms who sell such products find themselves quickly out of business. Some choices are not available because the government has established safety standards to which all products must conform. As chapter 2 shows, food safety legislation has provided federal agencies with broad authority to establish standards for fresh and processed foods. But are these regulations necessary? Can the unregulated market provide the level of food safety consumers are willing and able to pay for?

This chapter considers the efficiency of the unregulated market for food safety. The purpose of this chapter is to ascertain how product markets, with the particular characteristics of food products, work according to economic theory. By obtaining an understanding of how these markets work, we can gain insight into the situations in which the market can provide the level of food safety demanded by consumers. This understanding then provides the basis for considering whether government intervention in these markets can improve the efficiency of the unregulated market.

The Meaning of Safety

Safety means the absence of risk. Risk, in turn, is defined in decision theory with respect to characteristics of the probability distribution of an outcome such as contracting a disease. In a simple two-outcome case—a person is either healthy or sick—the higher the probability of contracting a food-borne disease, the greater the risk. Probabilities are numbers between zero and one, so

$$\text{safety} = 1 - \text{risk} = 1 - (\text{probability of disease}).$$

Thus, if eating meat that is known to be contaminated with *E. coli* conveys a 100 percent probability of illness, the meat is said to be unsafe or to be associated with a zero degree of safety. Conversely, eating meat that is known with a 100 percent probability to be uncontaminated is 100 percent safe.

According to this definition, safety is a relative concept. One action may result in a 50 percent probability of a minor illness, and another may result in a 50 percent probability of death. The severity of the outcome is not conveyed by the degree of safety. In decision theory the severity of risk is reflected in the maximum amount of money that people are willing to pay to avoid it or to insure against it. This amount is known as the person's risk premium. Each person's risk premium depends on his or her attitude toward risk, or degree of risk aversion. People exhibit different degrees of risk aversion and consequently may behave differently when faced with the same objective risk.

These concepts of safety and risk are different from those in the literature on toxicological risk assessment.

The objective of toxicological risk assessment is to establish a threshold dose of a toxicant below which adverse health effects are expected to be small or nonexistent. The connection between safety and toxicological risk assessment is the probability distribution of being exposed to a toxicant at or above the threshold level. If the probability of exposure above the threshold level is zero, safety is 100 percent.

The Demand for Food Safety

There are several theoretical approaches to the analysis of the demand for products differentiated by quality (for example, Hanneman 1982; Smith 1991; Smallwood and Blaylock 1991). Here we examine the demand for food safety by using the household production model of consumer demand in the health economics literature (Cropper and Freeman 1991; Antle and Capalbo 1994).

Let us define the household's objective as utility maximization, with the utility function depending on consumption goods, leisure time, and health status. The household produces consumption goods with purchased commodities, such as food and energy, and with household members' time. The health status of household members depends on their behavior (nutrition, occupational and incidental exposure to toxins, etc.) and on their predetermined physical characteristics. The household's behavior is constrained by its income and by its available time.

The demand for food with safety attributes derives from the disutility caused by illness and by the costs that illness imposes on the household. These costs are forgone work and leisure time while a household member is ill and medical expenses. Because the household receives higher utility when its members are healthy, it is willing to pay for safer and more nutritious foods that are associated with better health.

Several features of this model of food safety demand are important in the analysis of the market. First, the simple textbook theory of consumer demand is based on the assumption that consumers have perfect information about all products on the market. Yet many food product markets are characterized by imperfect information, a point discussed in detail below. Second, the theory requires that consumers know how product characteristics affect their health and well-being. Yet we know that some consumers may not be well informed about the relationship between product attributes and food safety. Third, the standard model assumes that all households have the same preferences of consumption, leisure time, and health. Preferences presumably differ across consumers; when health risk is involved, consumer perceptions often appear to differ substantially from prevailing scientific opinion. This point is illustrated by the contentious debate over the health effects of using recombinantly derived bovine somatotropin (rBST) in dairy production, where a wide range of knowledge about rBST and attitudes toward it have been expressed in consumer opinion surveys (Douthit 1991; Preston, McGuirk, and Jones 1991). Therefore, in the analysis of the market for food safety, we need to consider how the market functions under a variety of assumptions about consumer knowledge and behavior (for a related review of the literature, see Bockstael, Just, and Teisl 1994).

Supply and Market Equilibrium

Generally a high degree of safety costs more to produce than a low degree of safety. Competitive firms are willing to supply consumers with safety attributes they demand as long as the firms are remunerated for the cost of producing them. Consequently product differentiation by nutritional and safety characteristics in the food industry is important. In the 1980s food manufacturers began to put health claims on food labels, and in 1987 the FDA issued guidelines for claims that had previously not been allowed. Caswell and Johnson (1991) describe the kinds of product differentiation efforts that ensued by food manufacturers. A key issue in the behavior of both consumers and firms, therefore, is the availability of information about product characteristics.

The Role of Market Information. The textbook theory of competitive markets assumes that consumers and firms possess perfect information about prices and products in the market. But clearly information is costly and imperfect in many markets. By imperfect information we mean that all attributes relevant to the value of the product are not known. Stiglitz (1989) reviews the literature on product markets with imperfect information. This literature shows that the properties of market equilibrium depend on the characteristics of the product, on the cost of communicating information among consumers, and on the ability of consumers to use information.

One way to look at the issue of product quality is to ask under what conditions the market will provide the degree of quality that consumers want to purchase. When information about product quality before the purchase is imperfect, then consumers are put in the position of buying a product whose quality is uncertain. Firms could offer a product with a higher price to reflect its higher quality, but this raises a theoretical problem. If price is used by firms to communicate quality to consumers, then how will the process of competition work while consumers seek out the lowest price (Stiglitz 1989)?

In their seminal contribution Klein and Leffler (1981) provide a resolution to this paradox. They ask under what conditions will the unregulated market assure contractual performance, in the sense that firms will provide the product quality that consumers believe they are buying. They argue that as long as a substantial number of

41

knowledgeable consumers in the market demand a high-quality product and are willing to pay for it, the higher price is sufficient to ensure that nonperformance (supplying an inferior product) results in a loss greater than the gain from nonperformance. Price in such a market equals minimum average cost, where minimum average cost includes conventional average production costs plus the costs to the firm of establishing its reputation for supplying high quality. Klein and Leffler refer to this latter cost as the cost of investing in "brand-name capital." We refer to it here as the cost of establishing a firm's quality reputation.

For the purposes of our discussion of information about attributes of food quality, it is useful to distinguish several different types of information.

- *Perfect information.* Both seller and buyer have perfect information about the product. This is the assumption used in the textbook model of a competitive market. In the food safety area, this would be the case when a seller credibly reveals product quality to consumers or when consumers can ascertain quality from examination of the product before purchase. A consumer, for example, can see whether there are worm holes in an apple before buying, or a grocery store sells horticultural products that it certifies to be grown organically, or the manufacturer of a genetically engineered vegetable with a longer shelf life markets the product with a brand name (such as Calgene's Flavr Savr tomato).

- *Asymmetric imperfect information.* Information is perfect for the firm but imperfect for the consumer. This would be the case if a firm knew it applied a pesticide to a crop but the consumer cannot perceive the residues. It is important for the determination of market equilibrium in this case to observe, however, that even though the consumer's information may be imperfect before purchase, the consumer may realize quality after purchase.

A consumer who becomes acutely ill from a pesticide residue on a fresh fruit, for example, may realize the source of the illness. ~ *then what do they do?*

- *Symmetric imperfect information.* In this case information is imperfect for consumer and producer before and after purchase. This is typically the case of a food-borne disease transmitted through meat, as neither the firm supplying the product nor the consumer is aware that the meat is contaminated. As in the asymmetric information case, the consumer may or may not realize the source of the contamination after the fact. In some cases of food-borne illness, for example, symptoms such as diarrhea are immediate, and the consumer identifies the contaminated food as the source. In other cases, such as parasitic infections, symptoms are delayed, and consumers may not have any way to identify the source of the illness or to distinguish it from other types of disease.

The literature has identified three categories of goods according to the way consumers obtain information about them (Nelson 1970; Caswell and Padberg 1992; von Witzke and Hanf 1992). Search goods are those for which consumers have perfect information before purchase; experience goods can be judged only after purchase; and credence goods are those whose quality cannot be judged even after purchase. Thus, both experience goods and credence goods correspond to cases of imperfect information, either asymmetric or symmetric, because their definition does not consider the type of information available to the firm. As we see in chapter 4, the distinction between asymmetric and symmetric imperfect information plays a key role in the analysis of efficient regulation.

Properties of Market Equilibrium

Combining the key elements of the demand and supply sides of the market, the properties of market equilibrium can be analyzed. We consider the following cases: perfect information equilibriums; imperfect information when consumers realize quality after purchase; imperfect information when consumers cannot discern quality after purchase; heterogeneous consumer risk preference, production costs, and incomplete markets; and consumer knowledge of safety.

Perfect Information Equilibriums. Some food safety qualities are detectable by sight, smell, or touch—that is, by organoleptic inspection. Firms may declare a food's qualities, as in branded, genetically altered foods with desirable nutritional or safety qualities. In these cases the consumer may have nearly perfect safety information.

Even though food products may be differentiated by safety and nutritional characteristics, a competitive market can exist for the product as long as the standard conditions supporting competition exist. In the ideal case of perfect information, identical informed consumers, and free entry for identical, competitive producers, the perfectly competitive market functions efficiently. It provides consumers with the product they demand at minimum average cost of production.

When competitive firms are able to produce products with different levels of safety, then the marginal cost of safety will be equated with the marginal benefit of safety in competitive equilibrium, as illustrated in figure 3–1. This is the sense in which the competitive market achieves the "right" level of safety. It provides just as much safety as consumers are willing and able to buy.

The shapes of the marginal benefit and marginal cost curves in figure 3–1 have important implications for behavior and for efficient policy. If safety were costless, everyone would want perfect safety. But because safety is costly, perfectly informed, rational consumers generally choose less than 100 percent safety. One of the important policy implications is that regulations striving to

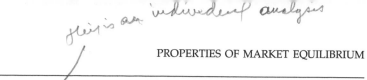

this is an individual analysis

FIGURE 3–1

MARKET EQUILIBRIUM DETERMINATION OF SAFETY

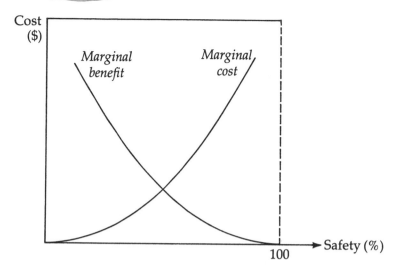

achieve zero risk are misguided on two counts. Zero risk is rarely achievable at any cost. Even if zero risk were achievable, it is rarely desired by individuals who know the true benefits and have to pay the costs of achieving it.

Few product markets meet the conditions of the perfectly competitive market, but many approximate them well enough to result in an efficient allocation of resources. But important violations of the perfectly competitive conditions may result in an inefficient level of safety. We now consider those violations of the perfectly competitive market model and discuss their effects on market equilibrium.

Imperfect Information When Consumers Realize Quality after Purchase. Imperfect information means that consumers lack perfect quality information before they purchase a product. But when consumers realize the

45

quality of the product after purchase, reputation can play an important role in determining the property of market equilibrium. This is typical of acute illness from toxic residues or of food-borne disease contracted immediately after consumption. If consumers buy the product repeatedly, firms that provide a higher quality (more safe) product can charge a higher price for it, and the market with imperfect prepurchase information can achieve the same outcome as the market with perfect information. When consumers purchase a product only once, an efficient equilibrium can also be attained as long as consumers can exchange product information or otherwise obtain product information at low cost. Here again firms can establish a reputation for a high-quality product and charge a commensurately high price to cover the cost of producing the product and establishing its quality reputation.

Many food markets satisfy the conditions that allow firms to establish quality reputations. Repeat purchases are typical of virtually all households' demand for food that is consumed at home. Moreover, low-cost information about product quality is available by word-of-mouth, newspapers, consumer information publications, and so forth. In addition, the rise of fast-food chains has made repeat purchases typical for food consumed outside the home, whether these purchases are made where one lives or on a trip. One of the most serious problems international travelers face is obtaining food and drink that meets their safety and quality expectations. The movement of many food service firms into international markets means that travelers can obtain a product with a known quality.

Imperfect Information When Consumers Cannot Discern Quality after Purchase. Consumers are usually not able to know product quality either before or after purchase when quality involves the chemical composition of the food, contamination with toxic chemicals, or the presence of microorganisms. Whereas acute effects of chemical contamination may be associated with the food source, the chronic effects of low-level exposure to toxins, such as cancer-causing substances, are difficult to know because the effects are delayed for many years or even decades. Moreover, because the causes of cancer and many other diseases are not well understood, it is difficult for consumers to associate exposure to any particular substance with the disease. Some acute effects of toxins or food-borne illness also occur with enough delay that consumers may not be able to associate the disease with the consumption of a contaminated food. Consumers also typically cannot discern quality that is related to the production process, as when food is irradiated or milk is produced with animals treated with genetically altered growth hormones such as rBST.

Under these conditions it is difficult for firms to establish reputations for quality, and the distinction between asymmetric imperfect information and symmetric imperfect information becomes important. With the latter the firm itself does not know all the quality attributes and so cannot reveal them even if it wants to or is required to do so by law. As the discussion of policy options in chapter 4 reveals, this difference plays a role in designing appropriate policies when the market fails to achieve the efficient degree of safety.

Clearly, when consumers cannot distinguish low-quality from high-quality products, the reputation mechanism cannot work effectively to achieve an efficient level of safety. Consequently, a Gresham's law of product quality applies, with "bad" (low-quality, low-cost) products chasing "good" (high-quality, high-cost) products out of the market. Thus, under these conditions the market fails to provide consumers who want a high-quality, safer product with the opportunity to buy it.

Heterogeneous Consumer Risk Preferences, Production Costs, and Incomplete Markets. Even when information is perfect, competitive markets may not provide the variety of quality and safety desired by all consumers. The market for food safety may be incomplete in this sense, but this incompleteness need not necessarily represent an inefficient allocation of resources in the economy.

As an example, consider the provision of products with a high degree of perceived safety, such as "organic" produce grown without pesticides. In many markets in the United States, such produce is available from firms that have established reputations for it sale. But in many other markets organically grown produce is not available. Undoubtedly some people in those markets would buy such products if they were available. Should we conclude that there is a market failure by virtue of the incompleteness of the market? To answer this question, it is necessary to understand how the market supplies safety-differentiated products. This requires an analysis of both demand and supply sides of the market.

People's attitudes toward risk appear to differ substantially. There are many examples of different behavior toward risk under similar degrees of risk information. Despite ample warnings about the risks of food-borne disease, for example, some people choose to eat uncooked or rare cooked meats and seafood while others do not.

Another factor that may explain differences in behavior is revealed by the household production model that was discussed above. According to the model, people not only have to be informed about risks, they also have to know or believe that they are vulnerable to them or are exposed to them. This phenomenon may explain why people with a history of cancer in their family may exhibit extreme risk aversion to behavior associated with cancer risk, while people with no family history may discount such risks.

The cost of supplying safety characteristics also varies from product to product and plays a role in the market equilibrium outcome. In some cases the cost of differentiating products by safety characteristic may be low; in this instance firms will be able to tailor products to even small segments of the market. The concentration of an additive in a product, for example, can be readily varied in the production or processing of the product, or both taste and safety can vary with the degree of cooking. This situation is illustrated in figure 3–2A by the existence of a horizontal segment of the firm's average cost curve in the safety dimension (where safety is assumed to be defined in continuous terms). Even though in this case average cost may not vary significantly with the degree of safety, other attributes of the product, such as taste or cosmetic quality, may change.

In other cases, firms with fixed plant and equipment may be able to produce efficiently only one degree of safety because of economies of safety-specific capital, such as contamination detection devices in processing or pest management technology in the production process. Figure 3–2B illustrates the average cost curves for this case. Under these conditions, only one or a few qualities may be offered in the market, depending on the demand for safety.

On the demand side, risk preferences and vulnerabilities in a population of individuals can be described with a probability distribution. When the distribution of risk preferences is tightly concentrated about some central value such as the mode of the distribution, as in figure 3–3A, then competitive firms may be able to supply a product only with that modal degree of safety. Those consumers in the tails of the distribution, who would prefer either a higher or lower degree of safety, are not provided those product options. This situation is an ex-

FIGURE 3–2
AVERAGE COST OF SAFETY

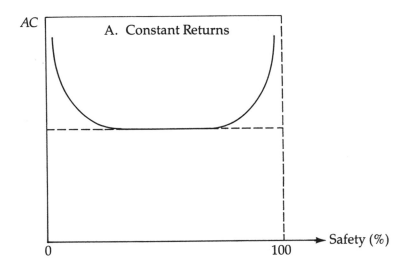

A. Constant Returns

Safety (%)

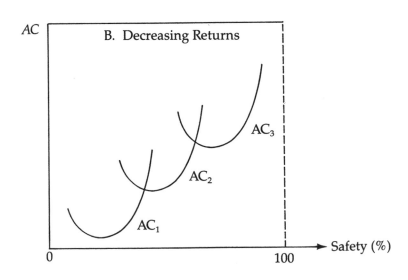

B. Decreasing Returns

AC_3

AC_2

AC_1

Safety (%)

FIGURE 3–3
DISTRIBUTIONS OF RISK ATTITUDES OR VULNERABILITIES IN THE CONSUMER POPULATION

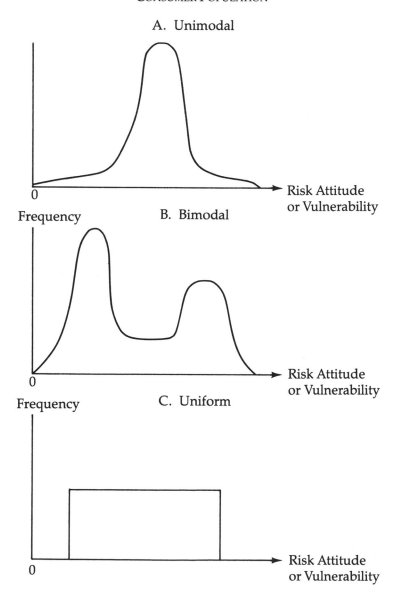

A. Unimodal

Frequency

Risk Attitude
or Vulnerability

B. Bimodal

Frequency

Risk Attitude
or Vulnerability

C. Uniform

Risk Attitude
or Vulnerability

ample of how heterogeneous preferences and costs of production may lead to incomplete markets. If the preference distribution is bimodal, as in figure 3–3B, the market may supply both low and high degrees of safety but not a middle value preferred by some consumers. If the preference distribution is uniform over a range of safety, as in figure 3–3C, and if a range of safety attributes can be produced at sufficiently low cost, it may be profitable for firms to provide an array of products with different safety qualities. The market may then be approximately complete with respect to degrees of safety demanded by consumers.

Let us now return to the question whether an "incomplete" market is an indication of an inefficiently functioning market. Clearly, when firms are supplying the variety of products that it is profitable to supply and there are no externalities in production or consumption that cause firms to undersupply, then the answer to this question must be no. In other words the market is providing as much variety in safety as is economical, and the market is therefore functioning efficiently.

There may well be cases, however, in which the market does fail to provide the desired variety of safety. Significant externalities, for example, may be associated with a communicable, food-borne disease. Consumers' demand for protection against the disease may be so low that they are not willing to pay for prevention, even though the collective net benefits from doing so would be positive.

Consumer Knowledge of Safety. By a knowledgeable consumer we mean one who is able to assess the quality attributes of a product if the information is available; a consumer lacking such knowledge is not able to assess product quality even if there is perfect quality information. Clearly, if none of the consumers were knowledgeable about food safety, there would not be a demand for safety. For most long-standing safety issues it can be assumed that there are many knowledgeable consumers, whereas most consumers may be unknowledgeable about new issues such as the use of rBST to raise dairy cow production. The risk preferences of the knowledgeable consumers also can be assumed to be heterogeneous. We assume that the distribution of risk preferences among the unknowledgeable consumers is the same as it is among the knowledgeable consumers.] *why?*

Under these conditions, competitive markets with symmetric perfect information, or with imperfect information and firm reputation, will provide an efficient level of safety for the knowledgeable consumers, for the reasons described above.

But what about the consumers who lack the knowledge to make use of product safety information? In the case of homogeneous risk preferences, the market will also be efficient, because the knowledgeable consumers will demand the degree of safety that the unknowledgeable consumers would want and the market will provide products with this degree of safety. This situation is analogous to the way markets respond to a majority of consumers who are informed about market price. A group of informed consumers is sufficient to ensure that all consumers receive a competitively priced product.

In the more realistic case of heterogeneous risk preferences, the market provides whatever safety characteristics are economically feasible given the distribution of risk preferences. The uninformed consumer is provided these options but does not know how to evaluate them in terms of safety and would have to select among them according to criteria other than safety, such as price. Given that unknowledgeable consumers select the product with the lowest price, and therefore the lowest quality, some will obtain less safety than they would if they were knowledgeable. Yet because the market does not *all bad choices means effic ??*

fail to provide consumers with choices, we cannot conclude that the market is inefficient.

B, S,

Conclusion

This chapter describes the characteristics of the market for food safety. A first finding is that efficient outcomes in the market for food safety can be obtained not only in the textbook case of a competitive market with perfect information but also in other important cases:

• When products are purchased repeatedly or low-cost product information is available and when consumers can ascertain product quality either before or after purchase, firms can establish reputations for product quality and charge a higher price for high-quality products.

• When a sufficient number of knowledgeable consumers exist, a demand for safety representative of the preferences of the larger population can be generated.

A second finding is that inefficient outcomes in the market for food safety can be obtained under several circumstances:

• when information is imperfect, consumers purchase a product only once, and information costs are high
• when information is imperfect for consumers both before and after purchase
• when a majority of consumers are unknowledgeable about product safety attributes

ah, what % is un ? 50%? 60%?

The principal results of this discussion are summarized in table 3–1. In three of the cases, the unregulated market achieves efficient equilibriums. Assuming that there is a relatively large proportion of the population that is knowledgeable about food safety reduces the number of inefficient cases to three. Additionally, many food purchases are characterized by repeat purchases or *where is the empirical evidence??*

TABLE 3–1
EFFICIENCY OF EQUILIBRIUMS IN THE MARKET FOR FOOD SAFETY

what about that those buying quality due to low quality (e.g. fresh salmon)

Product and Consumer Types		Type of Information	
	Perfect	Imperfect with quality realized after purchase	Imperfect with quality not realized after purchase
Repeat purchases or low-cost information	efficient	efficient	inefficient
Single purchases and high-cost information	efficient	inefficient	inefficient
Unknowledgeable consumers	inefficient	inefficient	inefficient

SOURCE: Author.

relatively low-cost information. Thus we can conclude that in all these cases economic theory predicts that the unregulated market is likely to meet the food safety demands of the public efficiently. Only when consumers' information is imperfect, both before and after purchase, is the market likely to fail to provide the desired degree of food product safety efficiently.

4
Principles and Tools for Efficient Food Safety Regulation

Chapter 3 shows that several key conditions may give rise to inefficient outcomes in the market for food safety. Imperfect information, incomplete markets, and uninformed consumers were identified as possible causes of market inefficiency. This finding indicates that there may be a role for government regulation to play in the market for food safety.

But saying that there *may* be a role for regulation does not mean that there *should* be regulation, nor does that premise tell us what form regulation should take when it is warranted. This chapter begins with a discussion of economic principles that should guide the design of food safety regulations, then discusses the policy options that are available and used in the food safety area, and concludes with a discussion of the cases identified in table 3–1.

Regulatory Principles

Principle 1. Food safety regulations designed to correct market failures are justified if, and only if, they pass a benefit-cost analysis test. This principle means that every regulation under consideration must be assessed for the benefits it generates relative to the unregulated market and for the costs it imposes on the economy. A necessary, but not sufficient, condition for adopting any regulation would be that it have a reasonable probability of generating positive net benefits.

To be meaningful, this principle requires that assessments of market failures be compared with the other real-world alternatives. It is not sufficient to argue that the market for food safety is characterized by imperfect information and therefore government regulation is called for. The market solution may not be the same as the perfect information equilibrium discussed in chapter 3, but it may nevertheless be more efficient than the feasible regulatory alternatives. More than two decades ago, Demsetz (1969) admonished those who would seek a regulation for every perceived market imperfection, and his message is relevant today:

> The view that now pervades much public policy economics implicitly presents the relevant choice as between an ideal norm and an existing "imperfect" institutional arrangement. This *nirvana* approach differs considerably from a *comparative institution* approach in which the relevant choice is between alternative real institutional arrangements. In practice, those who adopt the nirvana viewpoint seek to discover discrepancies between the ideal and the real and if discrepancies are found, they deduce that the real is inefficient. Users of the comparative institution approach attempt to assess which alternative real institutional arrangement seems best able to cope with the economic problem; practitioners of this approach may use an ideal norm to provide standards from which divergences are assessed for all practical alternatives of interest and select as efficient that alternative which seems most likely to minimize the divergence. (1)

Although the use of benefit-cost analysis in regulatory design is widely accepted by economists, it has not

57

been applied generally or consistently in the design of federal regulations. Until the Reagan administration, benefits and costs were explicitly considered in regulation making only if laws mandated it. President Reagan's executive order 12291 was the first comprehensive attempt to apply a general benefit-cost analysis test to all new federal regulations (Smith 1984). The Bush administration imposed a moratorium on new regulations and attempted to assess the efficiency of existing regulations. In 1993 President Clinton issued executive order 12866, which somewhat weakened the requirements of executive order 12291 but maintained the basic goal of requiring regulatory benefit-cost analysis for new regulations. According to the order, "Each agency shall assess both the costs and the benefits of the intended regulation and, recognizing that some costs and benefits are difficult to quantify, propose or adopt a regulation only upon a reasoned determination that the benefits of the intended regulation justify its costs."

More recently, there have been attempts to pass federal legislation that would require that regulations pass a benefit-cost test. Additionally, Representative Condit of California proposed an amendment to the 1994 USDA reorganization bill creating an office of risk assessment in the USDA and requiring risk assessments and benefit-cost analyses of regulations. The Clinton administration also is assessing the role that benefit-cost analysis should play in health and environmental regulation.

The requirement that regulations pass a benefit-cost analysis test can be given several interpretations and has important implications for regulation. First, applied to individual regulations, this principle would improve the efficiency of government regulatory activity by ruling out any regulation that is not reasonably expected to yield benefits in excess of its costs. As Smith (1984) observes, however, simply requiring that a regulation yield positive net benefits does not mean that a regulation is designed so that it *maximizes* net benefits.

Second, even though each regulation passes a benefit-cost analysis test, it does not follow that resources will be allocated efficiently across activities within a program or across program areas. When resources are constrained, all feasible regulations should be ranked by efficiency, with the most efficient ones being implemented until the budget is exhausted.

A third important implication of this principle is that, except in rare cases, policies that attempt to achieve a zero-risk standard will fail to pass the benefit-cost analysis test. As figure 3–1 illustrates, the marginal benefits of a higher degree of safety approach zero as safety approaches 100 percent, and marginal costs are typically high. Consequently, total costs typically exceed total benefits at some degree of safety less than 100 percent. Some advocates of health-based safety standards argue that the consideration of benefits and costs is wrong because it means that health and safety are being compromised. The fallacy in this argument is that whenever health-based regulations are promulgated, and thus regulatory resources are not efficiently allocated, federal agencies are in fact achieving less safety than they could with the resources that are available.

Benefit-cost analysis, like any complex analytical tool, can be used as well as abused. Regulatory decision making typically is a target of political influence and regulatory benefit-cost analysis can be distorted to serve the interests of the agency or political interests. Current law requires that the regulatory agencies conduct benefit-cost analyses themselves. These analyses must then pass the review of the Office of Information and Regulatory Analysis in the Office of Management and Budget, as well as be open to comment by private parties. Although in principle this process provides an extra-agency review, the public decision-making process would be better served if these analyses were produced by a credible, independent agency or entity.

Another critical problem in the food safety area is the treatment of uncertainties associated with health risks. The standard "conservative" health risk assessment procedures are also likely to create an inherent bias in favor of regulation (Nichols and Zeckhauser 1986). Our second principle addresses the problems of independence and uncertainty.

Principle 2. Regulatory benefit-cost analysis should be conducted independently of regulatory agencies and should provide comparable treatment of the uncertainties in benefit estimation and in cost estimation. The typical approach to benefit-cost analysis of a regulation is to assume that, without the regulation, external costs will be imposed on society because of market failure. A regulation designed to correct the failure therefore yields a benefit to society in the form of a reduction in the externality. The conventional analysis recognizes that there are costs of imposing regulations, typically in the form of administrative costs, as well as forgone benefits from higher production costs and reduced output in the regulated industry.

Consider the case of pesticide regulation under FIFRA. Health risks are estimated according to the established practice in toxicological risk assessment of including a safety factor to establish the RfD, or reference dose, which is considered to be safe. This reference dose is estimated with a safety factor ranging from 10 to 10,000, depending on the degree of uncertainty associated with the extrapolation of animal test results to humans (NRC 1993).

Yet there is no such standardized procedure for the use of uncertainty factors when the costs of regulations are estimated. There can be great uncertainty as to the potential economic costs of regulations. Besides the short-term impacts on production typically included in regulatory analyses, there are also potentially important long-term impacts of regulation on investment in research and development and on subsequent innovation.

As another example of how benefits and costs are often treated differently in regulatory benefit-cost analysis, consider the January 1994 regulatory impact analysis of the fish and seafood HACCP regulations proposed by the FDA. In this analysis, a range of benefits of the regulations was provided, based on a combination of expert opinion and modeling. Yet, on the costs side of the analysis, a single set of estimates was presented and was believed by external reviewers of the regulations to be unreasonably low and unrepresentative of the degree of uncertainty that existed in the estimates, as reported in the *Food Chemical News*, August 29, 1994.

Principle 3. Informed individual choice of safety is preferred to statutory safety standards when risk preferences are heterogeneous. If everyone in society has the same risk preferences, and if information is costly, the least-cost method of attaining the consensus degree of safety may be through legislation requiring that the standard be met by the industry. There is probably widespread agreement, for example, that the risk of contracting serious foodborne illnesses from fresh meats should be kept low. No one would want to buy meat labeled as contaminated with *E. coli* or *Salmonella*, but it is prohibitively costly for individuals to test for contamination. It may be efficient for government regulations to require that suppliers meet a minimum standard.

When preferences are heterogeneous, however, uniform standards are likely to be inefficient. In figure 3–3A a "fat tail" of the distribution goes toward zero. This tail indicates that some individuals in the population would prefer a lower degree of risk than the majority of the population, all else equal. But all else is not equal, namely, achieving a low degree of risk can be costly, as illustrated

61

in figure 3–1. Because of this heterogeneity in the population and the cost of producing safety, policy makers typically face difficult choices in setting standards. If they set standards high enough to encompass the preferences of most of the population, the regulations impose a higher degree of safety than many people would be willing to pay for. If regulators set standards to satisfy the average consumer, those who prefer a higher degree of safety, such as vulnerable individuals in the population, may be put at risk.

One of the most basic principles of economics is that imposing constraints on people's opportunities can only make them worse off. Thus, whenever there is substantial heterogeneity in risk preferences and people are informed about safety and health consequences of their choices, people will generally be better off choosing the level of safety they prefer rather than having to accept a uniform level of safety mandated by law. Thus, in the previous example, once a minimum standard is set to ensure that everyone receives a minimal degree of safety, those who prefer a higher degree of safety can choose it if the market provides that choice.

For example, choice is likely to be more efficient than uniform standards in the regulation of pesticide residues in foods. Restricting pesticide use in fruit and vegetable production raises their costs of production. The present regulatory regime, embodied in the Delaney clause of the Federal Food, Drug, and Cosmetic Act, imposes a zero-risk tolerance for pesticides that concentrate in processed foods. Alternatively, it would be possible to regulate pesticides to achieve a level of risk deemed to be minimal and to then allow foods that are produced without pesticides (so-called organic products) to be labeled as pesticide free. This alternative approach would be more efficient, as it would provide the minimal level of risk for which there is a consensus through a uniform regulation and would allow individuals who prefer a higher degree of safety to choose such foods without imposing the costs on everyone. An organic certification law was part of the 1990 farm bill and is being implemented. Unfortunately EPA's *de minimis* approach to pesticide regulation has been ruled inconsistent with the Delaney clause, as noted in chapter 2, and EPA's *de minimis* standard was unreasonably conservative.

Principle 4. Performance standards and incentive-based regulation are more efficient than design standards. The past twenty years of environmental and health regulation have taught important lessons about the inefficiency of some types of regulations. In particular, economists now understand that command-and-control regulation—the imposition of design standards on a production process to achieve regulatory goals—can be notoriously inefficient. Economists are critical of command-and-control regulation because "regulators generally lack the detailed knowledge of individual production facilities and processes and of alternative production and abatement methods that would be necessary to implement an efficient regulatory program" (Council of Economic Advisers 1990).

Thus process standards are particularly ill-suited to industries where process innovations are rapid. Command-and-control regulation discourages firms from innovating because of the costs involved in obtaining approval for new processes and because innovations may beget yet tighter regulatory standards. This is a particularly serious flaw in an industry such as food processing, where rapid innovation is occurring in many aspects of science and technology related to the detection and control of food-borne pathogens and toxicants. It may not be coincidental that the National Research Council's assessment of meat inspection procedures used by the USDA's Food Safety Inspection Service found that "the failure to apply sufficiently modern techniques to detect abnormalities in organs and tissues necessitates more extensive, yet less efficient, human resources during inspection" (NRC 1985, 9).

The principal example of command-and-control regulation in food safety is the FDA's use of good manufacturing practices that prescribe processes that must be used in food-processing facilities. The proposed mandating of HACCP systems in meat, poultry, and seafood inspection would represent a significant increase in the use of design standards in the food industry. The one existing mandated HACCP system was designed for control of botulism in the low-acid canned food industry. In that case the FDA provided specific instructions about types of equipment to be used and steps to be followed in preparing the food, filling the can, thermal processing, and evaluating the can seams (Pierson and Corlett 1992). In other industries, where production facilities vary significantly in scale, design standards are likely to be particularly inefficient, and their costs are likely to force small producers out of business.

Why Do Food Technologists Believe in Design Standards? There is a strong presumption among the scientific community working in the food safety field that process design standards are more efficient than performance standards. One explanation for this belief is the idea that testing for compliance to performance standards is expensive. This is true in some cases and not in others, but the relevant question is, expensive compared to what? The relevant comparison in this case is to the design standards. The problem here is that testing costs are explicit and easily known, whereas the costs of design standards are often not explicit. Whether expensive or not, at least some end-product testing is required to assure that design standards are working, a fact often ignored by the advocates of design standards. Note the requirement of verification in principle 6 of the HACCP system outlined in chapter 2.

64

A second argument for design standards is that the detection of diseases and other hazards that occur infrequently requires a high sample rate, and therefore destructive product testing is prohibitively expensive. Again, expensive compared to what? This argument also ignores that in many cases destructive testing is not required (that is, the testing of unpackaged meat or produce). This argument also reveals a misunderstanding of the purpose of performance standards and associated penalties for noncompliance. It is easily demonstrated that penalties sufficient to induce compliance with a performance standard can be calculated with available data. The penalties or fines for noncompliance (F) must be set so that the cost of production while not complying (C_{nc}) plus the expected penalty exceeds the cost of production under compliance (C_c). The expected penalty equals the probability of detection of noncompliance P times the penalty. Thus, it follows that an effective penalty must satisfy $F > (C_c - C_{nc})/P$. This formula implies that penalties for compliance must be higher, the higher is the cost of production under compliance, and the lower is the probability of detection. Thus, in cases where food-borne diseases and other contaminants are not likely to be detected frequently by testing, penalties must be set high enough to ensure compliance with the performance standard.

There are two valid reasons why performance standards may not be used: (1) end-product tests for safety are simply not available and (2) when contamination occurs at various stages of the production, processing, and marketing system, it can be costly to identify the source of the contamination. Both factors imply the potential benefits that could be obtained from research to develop better end-product tests, as well as from better technologies and information systems to track products throughout the production system (Roberts and Smallwood 1991). Emerging genetic methods may provide efficient

TABLE 4–1

APPROACHES TO THE CONTROL OF RISK

How Initiated	When Applied	
	Ex ante	Ex post
Private	injunction	liability
State	corrective tax, statutory regulation	fine for harm done

SOURCE: Shavell (1987).

means for identifying sources of disease at various stages of production.

Policy Tools for Food Safety Regulation

We now consider the policy tools that are available for food safety regulation. Shavell's (1987) classification scheme for approaches to the control of risk is presented in table 4–1. All four approaches are used to some degree in the food safety area, although the principal approach is statutory safety standards to prevent harm ex ante. Ex post liability for harm done is also an important factor in the regulation of health and safety. The following discussion considers the extent to which it may substitute or complement statutory regulation.

Statutory Regulation. Most food safety regulation in the United States takes the form of statutory regulation. Statutory regulations may take a variety of forms, each of which may have significantly different economic implications.

Public information and education. Chapter 3 describes the types of information imperfections that occur in food safety markets. Legislation may be designed to require firms to provide information to consumers, as in the case of nutrition labeling and product ingredient requirements. More generally, it would be possible to devise labels that present safety information. An example in the United States is the recent regulation by the USDA requiring labels on raw meats and poultry that provide information about safe handling and cooking. Another example is the color-coded safety labels for pesticide containers devised by the World Health Organization and used in many countries.

Firms may also be required to provide product safety information to government agencies, as in the case of pesticide registration under FIFRA or the approval of food additives under FFDCA. Similarly, public agencies may be charged with responsibility to conduct research to obtain information and to disseminate it to the public, as in various consumer education activities of the USDA and the FDA, land-grant university agricultural experiment stations, and cooperative extension programs.

Command-and-control regulation through design standards. As noted, this system of statutory or administrative rules requires the use of specific control devices or procedures to achieve regulatory goals. A principal tool of the FDA's regulation of food processing is the issuance of good manufacturing practice regulations that are a type of design standard for processing plants. Proposed mandatory HACCP systems for meat, poultry, and seafood inspection also would be design standards.

From an analytical point of view, the inefficiency of design standards is illustrated by simply observing that firms generally seek to implement the capital and operating procedures that minimize the cost of production. In the case of producing a product y with safety s, using input prices w and production technology t_p, the firm's cost function is $c(y, s, w, t_p)$. The general experience with design standards in environmental regulation is that when the government imposes a production technology t_g, $c(y, s, w, t_p) < c(y, s, w, t_g)$. In words, the firms' costs of producing a given product with given safety attributes are higher under the design standard than when the firms are allowed to choose the technology themselves.

Performance standards and incentives. Legislation can also establish food safety standards that must be met by final products. The most famous example in the food safety area is the zero cancer risk standard for pesticides embodied in the Delaney clause of FFDCA. In most cases, statutes do not state standards, and they are established through agency rule making, as in the EPA's 1985 interpretation of the Delaney clause as a *de minimis* standard of a one-in-one-million lifetime cancer risk. Another example of a performance standard is the recent decision by the USDA to impose a zero-tolerance standard for fecal contamination of poultry in processing plants. Another interesting example of performance standards and incentives is the establishment of allowable levels of bacterial and drug contamination in milk, with price incentives to producers who do not meet these standards (Caswell, Roberts, and Lin 1994).

Performance standards are generally believed by economists to be more efficient than command-and-control regulation in achieving a given standard. This gain in efficiency is attained because regulators who lack firm-specific information do not impose inappropriate design standards or try to micro-manage production processes. Instead, regulators monitor firms' performance to ensure that standards are met.

Following the preceding discussion of design standards, the analytical representation of the performance standard is that firms choose inputs and technology to minimize the cost of production $c(y, s, w, t_p)$, subject to the rule that the safety of the product, s, must meet or exceed the government standard s_g. If the firm does not meet the performance standard, it must pay a penalty imposed for noncompliance. As noted, a sufficiently high penalty must be imposed to guarantee compliance. The presumption of the superiority of performance standards over design standards is thus equivalent to the statement that $c(y, s_g, w, t_p) < c(y, s_g, w, t_g)$.

Both performance standards and command-and-control regulation, however, pose a fundamental problem: what standards should be set? Figure 3–1 demonstrates that as regulations attempt to achieve a higher degree of safety, the marginal cost of safety invariably rises, and both marginal and total costs of the regulations may become high. Consequently, at low degrees of risk, even small changes in standards may result in large changes in total costs of compliance (see, for example, Lichtenberg, Zilberman, and Bogen 1989). Unless standards pass a benefit-cost analysis test they are likely to be set too high. The zero-risk standard of the Delaney clause and the zero tolerance for fecal contamination in poultry mentioned are examples of unreasonably high standards.

Other forms of regulation can also have the effect of providing firms with incentives to produce products with desired safety attributes. The setting of a safety standard, for example, along with a third-party or government certification that a product meets the standard, may allow firms to market high-quality products that would otherwise not be profitable because of the imperfect information problem discussed in chapter 3.

Tort Liability. Legal scholars and economists recognize that tort law can be construed as a regulatory system. As table 4–1 shows, the tort law system involves privately initiated actions taken after harm has been done, in contrast to statutory regulation initiated by the state to prevent harm ex ante. Shavell (1978) identifies several conditions under which the tort system may prove effective: (1) when harm to an individual or a well-defined group is sufficient for the individual or group to have an incentive to sue the injurer for damages, (2) when injurers have sufficient resources to pay for the harm they cause, and (3) when individuals have information sufficient to demonstrate harm on an individual basis.

The economic theory of tort liability is based on the idea that the prospect of liability can induce firms (the potential injurers in cases of product liability) to take the socially optimal level of precaution that minimizes expected social cost associated with harm from a product. Define this expected social cost as the sum of the cost of taking precaution, $C(x)$, and the expected cost of an accident, $A(x)$. The optimal level of precaution that minimizes $C(x) + A(x)$ (assumed to be strictly convex in x) equates the marginal cost of precaution to minus the marginal expected cost of an accident. An efficient liability rule would induce firms to undertake precisely this level of precaution.

To some analysts, the attraction of the liability system as a form of regulation is its potential to achieve a higher level of efficiency than a statutory system. One of the fundamental problems with statutory regulation is the potential for regulators to impose uniform command-and-control standards that disregard differences among firms in their level of precaution, as well as differences among individuals in their demand for safety. Critics of statutory regulation point out that performance standards do not guarantee efficient regulation either. If performance standards do not have to pass a benefit-cost analysis test, they are likely to be set too high and thus to be inefficient relative to a tort liability system that did not set arbitrarily high standards.

The system of liability law in the United States has been strongly criticized as well (Huber 1988). The shift from common law based on contractual obligations—whether explicit or implicit—to the concept of strict liability is seen to result in a significant distortion of economic incentives. According to Huber,

The indiscriminate liability that characterizes modern tort law has done more than prevent the progress of safety: It has forced several great marches backward. The strategy of reducing liability by reducing effort and initiative across the board is all too common, and time and again one finds that safety itself is the largest casualty. (162)

In particular, Huber argues that the development of tort law discourages product differentiation according to safety characteristics, one of the features identified in chapter 3 as essential to the efficient functioning of the market for safety:

In all they did, the tort Founders and their followers were committed to a one-size-fits-all theory of safety and product defects. A small car was either defective or it was not; it did not matter in the least that a particular buyer might not be able to afford any other car and deliberately chose the compact as best for her needs and circumstances. In its single-minded assumption of uniformity, not just among products but among consumers themselves, the new tort jurisprudence proved to be a compulsive homogenizer. And that, in the most subtle but far-reaching way, undercut safety at every level. (167–68)

Other distortions of the legal system—such as the incentive for lawyers to undertake class-action suits that individuals would not undertake—could also lead to a higher degree of safety and less product variety than people want. According to economic logic, this excessive degree of safety could be the outcome of rational firms choosing to take more than the socially optimal level of precaution to avoid the risk of being sued.

Whether a liability rule can be economically more efficient than a statutory standard has been investigated in the economics literature but has not been resolved.

Shavell (1987) argues that liability is inefficient because some suits are never brought against injurers and because injurers do not need to defend against suits whose costs exceed the injurer's assets. Various other arguments have been leveled against liability, including the argument that the courts are technically incompetent to rule over health and safety issues (Viscusi 1984; Huber 1988). Rose-Ackerman (1991) argues that in a system based largely on statutory standards, the use of liability may actually be detrimental and that "real agencies are likely to perform better than awkward judicial hybrids that have many of the disadvantages of both forms." Litan (1991) reports that a set of studies conducted by the Brookings Institution shows that liability has not necessarily improved safety and may have actually discouraged innovation, although none of the examples come from the food industry.

Kolstad, Ulen, and Johnson (1990) demonstrate that under some conditions tort liability and statutory regulations can be complementary. Interestingly, some examples of hybrid laws have elements of both, as in the California Safe Drinking Water and Toxic Enforcement Act of 1986, under which standards are enforced through court cases that can be initiated by private parties or by state and local officials (Caswell and Johnson 1991). Innes (1994) goes even further and argues that with asymmetric information, as is typical with food safety, liability rules with appropriately set punitive damages can be designed to be more efficient than statutory standards. But whether the present system in the United States can accomplish this outcome remains an open question.

Finally, there is a somewhat irrational opposition to ex post regulation on the grounds that it is better to prevent harm than to react to it or to punish doers of harm after it has occurred. Consumer advocates, federal agency officials, and scientists appear to adhere to this view (for example, Crawford 1994). This argument seems to suggest a belief that ex ante regulation can achieve a zero degree of risk, and hence there is no reason to allow unregulated firms to do harm to consumers. This reasoning fails to recognize that zero risk is almost never attainable and that prevention can be motivated by the desire to avoid liability as much as by compliance with statutory safety standards.

Efficient Food Safety Regulation

We now consider how the principles discussed above lead to a choice of policy tools that would be best suited to the cases where the market may not be efficient, as identified in table 3–1. Recall that although table 3–1 is not an exhaustive delineation of situations that arise in food safety, it is representative of important cases. For the purposes of this discussion, we consider the following policy tools:

• *Product safety research and consumer education.* This category includes research on food safety knowledge and technology that are public goods and educational programs designed to convey food safety knowledge to consumers.

• *Product labeling requirements.* Firms are required to label products regarding their ingredients or any other characteristics that are deemed relevant to safety.

• *Safety performance standards that pass a benefit-cost analysis test.* Products marketed by firms are required to conform to standards of safety defined by law or by a regulatory agency.

• *Liability.* The design of rules regarding negligence or strict liability to allow private individuals or groups of individuals to seek compensation from harm caused by a firm's product through the courts.

Observe that command-and-control regulation is not included in the policy tool list, as it is ruled out by principle 4. If a statutory regulation is to be used, a performance standard is presumed to be more efficient than a command-and-control regulation.

Repeat Purchase Products or Single Purchase Products with Low-Cost Information. As table 3–1 shows, markets for these products are efficient when information is perfect and also when information is imperfect and firms can establish product quality reputation. These markets are inefficient when consumers are not able to discern product quality either before or after purchase, as with low levels of pesticide residues in foods. Consequently, reputation or low-cost exchange of information among consumers does not provide an incentive for firms to provide products with more than the minimal degree of safety that consumers can ascertain.

As long as consumers are knowledgeable about the use of food safety information, the obvious solution to the information problem is that firms be required to label products with information relevant to safety. Firms know what pesticides they have used in food production, for example, and some form of labeling could be devised, as has been done with nutrition labeling, to provide consumers with usable safety information. Viscusi (1993) discusses some issues that arise in product safety labeling. Consumers could choose among products with different price and safety attributes.

As Shavell (1987) notes, one situation in which safety standards are likely to be more efficient than liability is when consumers have difficulty knowing or proving harm ex post. Consumers do not know, for example, if the foods they eat contain pesticide residues, and they would have difficulty proving that chronic exposure to toxic chemicals in food caused cancer. Another relevant point is that even when consumers have heterogeneous safety preferences, there is likely to be a consensus for a minimal degree of safety. It follows, therefore, that a statutory minimum safety standard that passes a benefit-cost analysis test could be efficient. By also providing information to consumers in the form of required safety labeling, those consumers who preferred a higher degree of safety than the minimum could obtain it if such a market were economically feasible.

With symmetric imperfect information, neither the firm nor the consumer knows all a product's safety attributes. The seller of produce, for example, may know that certain pesticides are used in the production process but may not know whether residues are likely to be present in the product in sufficient amounts to pose a health risk. Clearly, such information about pesticides is a public good, and there is an inadequate incentive for individual firms to produce it. Thus there is also a role for public funding of research to generate health and safety information.

Single Purchase Products with High-Cost Product Quality Information. This is the example of the "tourist trap" restaurant. These markets are efficient with perfect information but inefficient with imperfect information. Because of the high cost of information about product quality, firms cannot establish quality reputations, and so the market equilibrium provides only low quality. Because health risks often involve acute effects, as with food-borne illnesses, firms are typically exercising some degree of precaution. In these situations, nonperformance is usually idiosyncratic and can be handled effectively through liability. A well-functioning liability law would induce an efficient level of precaution in these cases, except for firms with few assets, in which case it may be necessary to require that firms have liability insurance. It might be argued, for example, that in the case of fresh meat, poultry, and fish products, liability would not be sufficient to ensure that small processing firms take adequate safety precautions, whereas larger firms would. If insurance markets for small firms are not functioning well, then the appropriate policy would be to correct the failure in the insurance market.

Consumer Knowledge of Food Safety. The most glaring fact in table 3–1 is that, regardless of information regime, the outcome is not efficient when most consumers lack knowledge of the safety attributes of a product. Even a well-functioning competitive market cannot make choices for people. Clearly, such knowledge is a public good, and therefore public consumer education is warranted. Publicly funded research can be justified to develop the knowledge that consumers need.

Despite educational efforts, some consumers may remain unable to make decisions for themselves or their families. Indeed, this is an issue much studied in the nutrition field (NRC 1990). Consumer ignorance is not an indication of an inefficiently functioning market but apparently is an important motivation for the paternalistic view that government is responsible for those who seemingly cannot take care of themselves. It can be argued that education, labeling, and liability rules are ineffective to protect these individuals; therefore statutory regulations should be invoked.

By principles 1 and 2 presented above, a performance standard designed to protect unknowledgeable consumers should pass a benefit-cost analysis test. The setting of an acceptable standard will depend on the number of consumers who benefit from the standard and the costs associated with the standard. As noted, one of the costs of a uniform standard is the taking away of choice from those informed consumers who would prefer a lower level of safety than is imposed by the standard. Without a standard the market provides the minimal degree of safety that knowledgeable consumers demand. A benefit-cost analysis can determine if more people would be made better off than worse off with a statutory standard.

Unknowledgeable consumers may tend to have lower levels of education and lower incomes than informed consumers. Thus, it might be tempting to argue that imposing a strict regulatory standard would represent an income transfer from high- to low-income households. But this conclusion is correct only if unknowledgeable consumers systematically prefer higher degrees of safety than other consumers. In fact we might expect just the opposite to be true because consumers who are highly risk averse have more of an incentive to be informed (Benjamin 1993). Thus, setting a strict standard would implicitly transfer income from individuals who prefer a lower degree of safety, whatever their income level, to individuals who prefer a higher degree of safety.

Conclusion

Four principles for efficient food safety regulation were identified:

1. Regulations must pass an independent benefit-cost analysis test.
2. Uncertainty associated with estimation of both benefits and costs of regulation must be treated consistently in regulatory benefit-cost analysis.
3. Individual choice is generally more efficient than uniform statutory risk standards.
4. Performance standards and incentive-based regulation are generally more efficient than mandatory design standards.

These principles were used to identify the efficient forms of regulation when the unregulated market is inefficient. The results of this analysis are summarized in table 4–2. For most cases, education, labeling, and liability are efficient solutions. Notably, even when consumers have imperfect quality information before and after pur-

TABLE 4–2
EFFICIENT POLICY TOOLS IN THE MARKET FOR FOOD SAFETY

Product and Consumer Types	Perfect	Type of Information		
		Imperfect with realization after purchase	Asymmetric imperfect without realization after purchase	Symmetric imperfect without realization after purchase
Repeat purchases or low-cost information exchange	market	market	labeling	performance standards
Single purchases and high-cost information exchange	market	liability	labeling	performance standards
Consumer lack of safety knowledge	education	education, liability	education, labeling	education, performance standards

SOURCE: Author.

chase of a product, product labeling requirements can solve the consumer's information problem as long as producers and sellers have quality information. The one class of problems where statutory regulation is indicated as possibly being the efficient solution is when *both* consumers and producers have imperfect information about product quality. In that case, firms cannot reveal quality information under a labeling law because they do not have it.

78

[handwritten margin notes:] empirically how ? * is this case ?

The farmer knows, but the grocery store does not know about pesticide in the crop.

5
Toward Regulatory Reform

Chapter 3 provided analysis of the efficiency of the unregulated market for food safety. Chapter 4 outlined principles for efficient regulation in those cases where market outcomes are not efficient. This chapter applies those analyses to assess the current regulatory system described in chapter 2. This assessment in turn provides the basis for recommendations for regulatory reforms.

Where Is Regulation Warranted?

Returning to the analysis of chapters 3 and 4, we can categorize food safety issues according to the information criteria summarized in tables 3–1 and 4–1.

A. *Perfect information.* Safety characteristics discernible by sight, touch, or smell, such as freshness, cleanliness, presence of fatty tissue, etc.; also when product quality is reliably identified by the producer or a third party, for example, branded genetically engineered products, or certified organic products.

B. *Imperfect information for consumers before purchase, quality realized after purchase.* Contamination by disease, chemicals, or physical objects that results in acute, recognizable effects when the food is consumed.

C. *Imperfect information before and after purchase for consumer, but perfect information for producer.* All process-related aspects of safety, for example, use of pesticides, use of genetically altered products in production, use of irradiation.

79

D. *Imperfect information before and after purchase for producer and consumer.* Food-borne diseases not readily identified in the production process, not readily identified by consumers as to food source because of delayed symptoms; low-level pesticide residues that cause chronic health effects; nutritional and safety characteristics of newly developed plant varieties.

The analysis of chapters 3 and 4 identified characteristics of food product markets that are likely to cause those markets to function efficiently in the provision of food safety quality. Two broad sets of conditions appear to be necessary for market efficiency:

- Firms must be able to establish reputations for quality and charge a price that reflects this quality.
- Enough consumers in the market must have the knowledge needed to evaluate safety attributes of foods.

Under these conditions, markets function efficiently without government regulation in cases A and B defined above and can function efficiently in case C with the requirement of safety and nutrition labeling that corrects the information imperfections in the market. Remarkably, then, economic analysis suggests that the majority of product markets can provide the efficient measure of food product safety with, at most, labeling requirements. When some consumers lack adequate knowledge of food safety, public education programs are also warranted.

In returning to the description of the existing system of food safety regulation, it is apparent that existing nutrition labeling and education policy is broadly consistent with this analysis. Rather than attempt to legislate what kinds of foods people eat, nutrition education efforts, such as those in the Nutrition Labeling and Education Act, are designed to complement labeling. Recent efforts by the USDA's Food Safety Inspection Service to utilize safety labeling and education also have emphasized the importance of consumer information and education in reducing the incidence of food-borne illness. The analysis presented in this study supports an expanded role for consumer research and education to develop safety labeling and education as a substitute for unnecessary and inefficient standards and design regulations implemented under FFDCA.

Chapter 2 indicates that most statutory food safety regulation under FFDCA is broadly *inconsistent* with the conclusions of the analysis in chapters 3 and 4. The food adulteration concepts of the act have led to a heavy reliance on design standards rather than on performance standards. Moreover, the provisions of sections 408 and 409 of FFDCA regarding food additives and the regulation of pesticides involve the imposition of zero-risk standards that are inconsistent with the economic analysis of efficient regulatory procedures.

The analysis of chapters 3 and 4 also indicates that there is one general set of conditions under which statutory safety standards may be required, namely, when both firms and consumers have imperfect information about product safety before and after purchase, that is, case D. These conditions correspond to the contamination of food with microorganisms, chemicals, and other hazards that are not readily tested for in the manufacturing process and that affected consumers cannot readily associate with a food source. Category D also would apply to the nutritional or safety characteristics of new varieties of foods developed by genetic engineering techniques.

Consistency with Regulatory Principles

Where regulation is needed, it should be consistent with the principles outlined in chapter 4. Here we consider each principle and the extent to which each major part of food safety legislation is consistent with it.

Consistency with principles 1 and 2. Regulations must pass an independent benefit-cost analysis test that considers equally the uncertainties in the estimation of the benefits and the costs of regulation. Food safety legislation in FIFRA and section 408 of FFDCA is generally consistent with the principle that regulations should pass a benefit-cost analysis test. These laws state that the risks should be balanced against the benefits of pesticides in pesticide registration and tolerance setting. Section 409's Delaney clause, however, is not consistent with this principle. But even where the risks and benefits should, in principle, be considered in pesticide regulation, principle 2 is violated by "conservative" estimation of health risks. Typically, worst-case assumptions are made at each stage in the risk estimation process, and arbitrary uncertainty factors are used in calculating reference doses. Moreover, the EPA, rather than an independent agency or party, is responsible for conducting the assessments of the benefits and costs, and this situation may lead to a bias in favor of regulation.

The 1994 legislative agenda contains several proposals to add benefit-cost analysis requirements across the board to all regulation making in the federal government, as well as within the USDA. Such provisions could represent a major step toward efficient regulation if they did not duplicate existing analyses and if they were implemented effectively. The experience with pesticide reregistration under FIFRA and the Bush administration's attempt at regulatory reform using executive order 12291 have both shown that it is not feasible to require that benefit-cost analyses be conducted for all existing regulations unless adequate resources are devoted to the task. Simply requiring that new regulations conform to more rigorous procedures may itself create some distortions by making more efficient regulations difficult to implement while older, less efficient regulations remain in place. Clearly, flexibility and judicious use of this tool is called for.

The importance of assuring that regulatory benefit-cost analyses be conducted independently cannot be overemphasized. Analyses performed by regulatory agencies can easily be distorted to yield the outcome desired by the agency. The recent example of the FDA's regulatory impact analysis of the fish and seafood HACCP regulations illustrates this point (FDA 1994a).

The Clinton administration's proposals for pesticide regulation reform would eliminate the benefit-cost aspects of FFDCA in section 408 and would replace it and the Delaney clause with a strict *de minimis* standard. The proposal to follow the NRC (1993) recommendation for pesticide tolerances for children could result in even more conservative estimation of toxicological risk and thus lead to lower tolerances and even fewer pesticides being registered for use. This change would be made without considering the costs of the regulations, for example, the resulting increased health risks to the general population from reduced consumption of fresh fruits and vegetables, as well as the economic costs of more strict pesticide restrictions. These aspects of the Clinton administration's proposal for pesticide regulation reform clearly are inconsistent with the principles for efficient regulation.

Many other regulations are being imposed without passing a benefit-cost test. Recently, for example, the USDA imposed a zero tolerance of fecal contamination of beef carcasses in slaughter houses to reduce the incidence of *E. coli* contamination. While reduction of *E. coli* contamination is a desirable goal, it is not obvious that this regulation is the most cost-effective way to achieve that outcome.

A related new regulation is USDA's announced goal of mandating newer, more rapid microbial testing in

83

meat and poultry processing. The meat industry opposes such testing and argues that other, less costly approaches are better. Again, without a benefit-cost analysis of these alternatives, it is impossible to know whether the proposed regulations are the best approach or not.

Consistency with principle 3. Whenever possible, rely upon individual choice of safety rather than statutory regulation. The existing approach to nutrition labeling and education is clearly consistent with this principle, although FDA's implementation of this approach is arguably too restrictive in some respects (Calfee 1994). Although both the FDA and the USDA have promoted research and education programs to improve consumers' knowledge of food safety, it is also clear that choice facilitated by education and labeling could replace statutory regulation and mandated process regulations in many instances. The current regulatory approach to food additives and meat inspection is based on the strong presumption that uniform levels of safety are the appropriate policy, that is, the "one size fits all" approach to safety. Yet variable standards and labeling could better tailor food safety choices to the varying needs of a diverse population.

A clear example where choice could play a role is pesticide regulation. The 1993 NRC report on pesticides in the diets of infants and children recommended that pesticide residue tolerances be set to account for the higher possible exposures and vulnerabilities of infants and children. The implication of this recommendation is that tolerances should be set *uniformly* higher to address this concern. As a result, some existing tolerances could be canceled, and some new pesticides could fail to be approved for some or all uses. An alternative approach would be to establish higher standards for those foods, such as fruit juices, that are consumed in large quantities by children, and to provide label information for those products that meet the higher standard. In this way, manufacturers of these products could charge a higher price for them, to the extent that they were more costly to produce, and consumers desiring this additional degree of safety could obtain it. At the same time, those not wanting or unable to afford that degree of safety would not have to forgo the nutritional benefits of those products.

A similar approach could be pursued in many other areas of food safety. In the control of food-borne diseases, for example, animals can be raised and processed under hygienic conditions so that the products can meet higher standards of safety and other aspects of quality such as fat content. Labeling these products as meeting specific safety or health standards then provides the conditions, as discussed in chapter 3, under which the market for safety can operate efficiently.

Labeling also has been debated for genetically engineered foods and drugs. Current FDA policy is not to require labeling of genetically engineered products on the basis of the principle that the end-product quality matters, not the process used to derive the plant variety. As described in chapter 2, the FDA has also issued guidelines for firms that want to market milk produced with cows that have not been treated with rBST. Generally, the principle outlined in chapter 3, that individual choice is preferred over uniform standards, is consistent with allowing labeling that is accurate and not misleading. With substantial uncertainty about the safety attributes of genetically engineered foods and other production processes, it makes sense to allow firms to provide accurate information about the process used. Consumers can then make a choice according to price and the various quality and safety attributes they associate with the product, including the process used to produce it. If indeed the process has no effect on safety, this fact will become clear over time, and superfluous process labeling will be rejected by the market. But the costs of marketing labeled products should be borne by the producers and consumers of those products, not by the general taxpayers through subsidized certification programs. The same principles should apply to the development of organic certification of foods under the provisions of the 1990 farm bill. Once the USDA has established reasonable criteria for organic certification, the costs of certification should be borne by the industry.

As Viscusi (1993) observes, product safety labeling should be a federal responsibility to avoid the costly proliferation of potentially inconsistent state labeling laws. The rBST labeling issue illustrates the tendency for this problem to arise, with some states disallowing all labeling regarding use of rBST, some states following FDA guidelines, and other states developing separate rules (chapter 2).

Another key point emphasized by Viscusi is the need to base safety labeling on a science-based risk communication strategy. State laws such as California's proposition 65 have mandated the use of arbitrary uncertainty factors in risk assessments in the same way the EPA incorporates them into assessments of pesticide cancer risk. Moreover, the California approach requires labels that do not effectively communicate the relative risks associated with different products. Research is needed to investigate how product safety labels could be designed to effectively convey the risk and safety information to consumers.

Consistency with principle 4. Performance standards and incentives are preferred to command-and-control regulation. Many aspects of existing food safety regulation rely upon process design standards rather than performance standards. The FDA, for example, mandates good manufacturing practices for processing facilities. The most sweeping move toward process design standards is the announced goals of both the FDA and the USDA to implement HACCP systems for all the food industry, including meat, poultry, and fish and seafood. In August 1994 FDA Commissioner Kessler announced that the move toward implementing HACCP systems represented "one of the broadest food safety policy shifts in the last 50 years."

As described in chapter 2, HACCP is a quality control system that uses risk assessment procedures to identify hazards and to establish "critical control points" for them. The degree to which HACCP becomes a strict process design standard depends on how federal agencies implement it. A federal agency could establish performance standards to be met at stages in the food production, processing, and marketing system, while allowing firms to decide how to meet those standards. Under this approach to HACCP, the federal government's role is limited to setting and monitoring standards.

Agencies are more likely to impose specific design standards that must be used as part of the HACCP system, as the FDA has done for the low-acid canned food industry. The HACCP for low-acid canned food involves thirty to forty critical control points (Pierson and Corlett 1992). Clearly, this design-oriented approach to HACCP would be less efficient than the performance-standard approach. A similar, mandatory approach based on design standards was proposed by the FDA for the fish products industry (FDA 1994b).

Another key problem with mandatory HACCP systems is that the hazards designated for control are presumed to be sufficiently important to justify the cost of control. But such a conclusion could not be drawn from the regulatory impact analysis conducted by the FDA for the fish and seafood HACCP, where all hazards to be controlled were analyzed together. Indeed, one of the criticisms by industry of the mandatory approach proposed by the FDA was that equally strict rules applied to the whole industry even though there is ample evidence that certain seafood products, such as shellfish, represent most of the risk.

Moreover, when critical control points are set (that is, the standards are set), there is no guarantee that they will be set efficiently. Indeed, statements of HACCP principles and guides for their implementation fail to give any consideration to the benefits versus costs of control. Thus, as typically constructed, mandatory HACCP systems could fail to pass a benefit-cost analysis test.

 Another important question about HACCP is whether it is more cost effective for the regulatory agency to impose and monitor standards at each stage of the production process, or only at the final product stage. Surprisingly, this basic question has not been carefully researched and was not addressed in the fish and seafood HACCP regulatory impact analysis. Once again, the presumption by scientists and regulators appears to be that design standards are the only appropriate means to achieve safe food.

Recommendations for Regulatory Reform

Based on the preceding assessment of the existing system of food safety regulation, we now propose recommendations for regulatory reform.

Recommendation 1. Undertake an independent, across-the-board assessment of priorities to determine whether research, education, and the various forms of regulation are being efficiently utilized, and how food safety regulatory activity of the federal government would be most efficiently organized. A number of consumer groups, industry representatives, and scientists argue that food safety regulation would be conducted more efficiently if all responsibilities were assigned to one agency. The single-agency model could facilitate the assessment of priorities and resource allocation across the various areas of food safety regulation. It does seem reasonable to ask whether it is time to consider consolidating the diverse laws and agencies that are involved in food safety regulation.

The single-agency model, however, has several problems. First, where does food safety responsibility end, and health, environment, and other areas of responsibility begin? Many areas of health and safety overlap. An additional question about the single-agency model is whether the assignment of all responsibilities to a single agency provides the correct incentives within the bureaucracy. It could be argued that a multiagency system of checks and balances would be better. As chapter 3 noted, independent rather than in-house benefit-cost analyses are needed because these analyses can be "cooked" by agencies to satisfy their agendas. This problem suggests a different, decentralized model for the redesign of food safety regulation, wherein legislation assigns responsibility for benefit-cost analyses to an independent agency or even an extragovernmental organization and also requires implementing agencies to allocate effort and resources accordingly.

Recommendation 2. A principal goal of food safety policies— research, education, and design of statutory standards— should be to enhance the capacity of producers and consumers to make informed safety choices. Specific recommendations follow:

• Research and education to support safe storage, handling, and cooking by consumers and food service workers.

• Research and education to improve knowledge about the linkages between diet, nutrition, and health.

• Research to develop criteria for safety labeling. Numerous questions need to be addressed to implement safety labeling. How should safety be integrated with nutritional considerations in design of labels? How can a system of variable safety standards and labeling replace the system of uniform standards? What types of safety concerns can be supported with this type of system?

• Development of safety labeling for products produced with new technologies when risk data indicate they are appropriate. Allowed use of new technologies with higher risks, subject to labeling requirements that indicate scientifically established risks. Technology approval rules to be revised to streamline the approval process for technologies that are considered low risk.

• Products labeled as certifiably produced by a process, with the costs of such certification borne by producers and consumers of those products (for example, brand-name labeling of foods genetically engineered for longer shelf life, improved nutritional content, or greater safety; labeling of products as organically grown without pesticides; labeling of dairy products as not produced with cows treated with rBST).

Recommendation 3. Where industrywide food safety performance standards are indicated as the most efficient regulatory approach—those cases where firms and consumers have imperfect safety information both before and after production and consumption of a food product—the standards should pass an objective benefit-cost analysis test.

• Replacement of the Delaney clause with a *de minimis* risk standard to be applied to all products, whether raw or processed. Pesticide registration should be allowed for those products that exceed *de minimis* risk if they pass a benefit-cost analysis test. Foods expected to contain higher than *de minimis* residue levels should be labeled accordingly.

• Research to support development of efficient performance standards and testing procedures.

• Development of integrated economic, medical, and biological data for risk assessments needed to set efficient standards.

- Research to compare the efficiency of HACCP systems to final product performance standards.
- Benefit-cost analysis tests for hazards to be controlled and for critical control points in HACCP systems.

Recommendation 4. Process design standards should be replaced by a system of performance standards and incentives.

- Development of safety standards and labeling to support product markets for safety-differentiated products.
- Research funding to support development of efficient standards and testing procedures for biological, chemical, and physical hazards: specifically, the integration of economic, disease incidence, and health data to support the identification of hazards for control.
- Definition of HACCP systems as performance standards at each stage of production, not as design standards.

Implications for the 1995 Farm Bill

Food safety has not been a principal objective of the 1990 farm bill or its predecessors. Whether the 1995 farm bill should do so is an open question. Advocates of an overhaul of food safety legislation, such as the Safe Food Coalition, would have all food safety regulatory authority assigned to one agency, such as the FDA. These consumer groups argue that food safety reform should assign responsibility for meat inspection to the FDA. According to this view, clearly, food safety legislation should not be incorporated into the 1995 farm bill. But unless such comprehensive food safety reform is undertaken and food safety responsibility is assigned to an agency other than the USDA, it seems appropriate to consider the degree to which the food safety policy reforms outlined above could fit into new farm legislation, perhaps as a food safety title. Several important aspects of needed reforms could be addressed in the 1995 farm bill.

Research. In some important areas, publicly funded research is needed to improve the science base for food safety education and to devise more efficient regulations such as those for safety labeling. Substantial capacity to conduct this research exists within the USDA, land-grant universities, private universities, and the private sector. To ensure that this research is performed on a competitive basis, a component of the national research initiative could be targeted to address the research questions in the food safety area.

Education. As emphasized above, consumer education is a critical aspect of an efficient approach to food safety policy. The farm bill could specifically direct cooperative extension to address needed food safety education to complement the Nutrition Labeling and Education Act of 1990.

Efficient Regulation. The recent USDA reorganization established an office within that agency to conduct benefit-cost analyses of the USDA regulations. Although the above recommendations are obviously consistent with the goal of subjecting the USDA's regulations to benefit-cost tests, there are several problems with the proposal to conduct these analyses within the USDA. First, the USDA's Economic Research Service has the capacity to conduct benefit-cost analyses and has done a number of such studies (for example, on ethanol policy, the Conservation Reserve Program). Second, as noted, regulatory benefit-cost analyses need to be done independently of implementing agencies to ensure objectivity.

References

Anderson, S. C. Letter to Richard A. Williams, Office of Scientific Analysis and Support, Food and Drug Administration, commenting on FDA's proposed fish and seafood HACCP regulations. May 31, 1994.

Antle, J. M., and S. M. Capalbo. "Pesticides, Productivity, and Farmer Health: Implications for Regulatory Policy and Agricultural Research." *American Journal of Agricultural Economics* 76 (August 1994): 598–602.

Archibald, S. O., and C. K. Winter. "Pesticides in Our Food: Assessing the Risks." In *Chemicals in the Human Food Chain*, edited by C. K. Winter, J. N. Seiber, and C. F. Nuckton. New York: Van Nostrand Reinhold, 1990.

Barefoot, S. F., R. N. Beachy, and M. S. Lilburn. *Labeling of Food-Plant Biotechnology Products*. CAST Issue Paper 4. Ames, Iowa, July 1994.

Becker, G. S. "HACCP: Prescription for Safer Food or Smokescreen for Deregulation?" *Choices*, 2d qtr. 1992, pp. 28–29.

Benjamin, D. K. "Risky Business: Rational Ignorance in Assessing Environmental Hazards." In *Taking the Environment Seriously*, edited by R. E. Miners and B. Yandle. Lanham, Md.: Rowan and Littlefield, 1993.

Bockstael, N. E., R. E. Just, and M. F. Teisl. "Food Safety and Inspection: An Overview." In *Re-engineering Marketing Policies for Food and Agriculture*, edited by D. I. Padberg. Proceedings of the Food and Agricultural Marketing Consortium, Alexandria, Va., January 1994.

Calfee, J. E. "Worried about Your Health? FDA Isn't." *Wall Street Journal*, September 12, 1994.

Caswell, J. A., ed. *Economics of Food Safety*. New York: Elsevier Science Pub. Co., 1991.

Caswell, J. A., and G. V. Johnson. "Firm Strategic Response to Food Safety and Nutrition Regulation." In *Economics of Food Safety*, edited by J. A. Caswell. New York: Elsevier Science Pub. Co., 1991.

Caswell, J. A., and D. I. Padberg. "Toward a More Comprehensive Theory of Food Labels." *American Journal of Agricultural Economics* 74 (May 1992): 460–68.

Caswell, J. A., T. Roberts, and C. T. J. Lin. "Opportunities to Market Food Safety." In *Food and Agricultural Markets: The Quiet Revolution*, edited by L. P. Schultz and L. M. Daft. Washington, D.C.: ERS/USDA and National Planning Association, 1994.

Council for Agricultural Science and Technology. *Pesticides: Minor Uses/Major Issues*. Ames, Iowa: CAST, June 1992.

Council of Economic Advisers. *Economic Report of the President, 1990*. Washington, D.C.: U.S. Government Printing Office, 1990.

Crawford, L. M. "Emerging Issues in Food Safety." *Health and Environmental Digest* 7 (March 1994): 11–13.

Cropper, M. L., W. E. Evans, S. J. Berardi, M. M. Ducla-Soares, and P. R. Portney. "The Determinants of Pesticide Regulation: A Statistical Analysis of EPA Decision Making." *Journal of Political Economy* 100 (February 1992): 175–97.

Cropper, M. L., and A. M. Freeman III. "Environmental Health Effects." In *Measuring the Demand for Environmental Quality*, edited by J. B. Braden and C. D. Kolstad. Amsterdam: North-Holland, 1991.

Demsetz, H. "Information and Efficiency: Another Viewpoint." *Journal of Law and Economics* (April 1969): 1–22.

Douthit, R. A. *Recombinant Bovine Growth Hormone: A Consumer's Perspective*. Madison, Wisc.: Robert M. La Follette Institute of Public Affairs, 1991.

Fisher, L., and D. D. Haley. "Joint Statement of Linda Fisher, assistant administrator for pesticides and toxic substances, Environmental Protection Agency, and Daniel D. Haley, administrator, Agricultural Marketing Service, U.S. Department of Agriculture, before the Committee on Agriculture, Nutrition, and Forestry, United States Senate." June 5, 1991.

Fleisher, B. "The Economic Risks of Deliberately Released Genetically Engineered Microorganisms." *American Journal of Agricultural Economics* 71 (May 1989): 480–84.

Food and Drug Administration. "Statement of Policy: Foods Derived from New Plant Varieties." *Federal Register* 57 (1992): 22984–23005.

Food and Drug Administration. "Preliminary Regulatory Impact Analysis of the Proposed Regulations to Establish Procedures for the Safe Processing and Importing of Fish and Fishery Products." January 24, 1994a.

Food and Drug Administration. "Proposal to Establish Procedures for the Safe Processing and Importing of Fish and Fishery Products; Proposed Rule." *Federal Register*, January 28, 1994b: 4142–14.

Food and Drug Administration. "Food Safety Assurance Program; Development of Hazard Analysis Critical Control Points; Proposed Rule." *Federal Register*, August 4, 1994c: 39888–96.

Forsythe, K., and P. Evangelou. "Costs and Benefits of Irradiation Quarantine Treatments for U.S. Fruit and Vegetable Imports." In *Environmental Policies: Implications for Agricultural Trade*, edited by J. Sullivan. U.S. Department of Agriculture, Economic Research Service, Foreign Agricultural Economic Report 252, June 1994.

Francis, F. J. *Food Safety: The Interpretation of Risk*. Ames, Iowa: Council for Agricultural Science and Technology, April 1992.

Gantz, H. "The Nation's Food Protectors: Who Are They? What Do They Do?" *Food News for Consumers*, Winter 1990, 4–5.

Hallberg, M. C., ed. *Bovine Somatotropin and Emerging Issues: An Assessment*. Boulder: Westview Press, 1992.

Hanneman, W. M. "Quality and Demand Analysis." In *New Directions in Econometric Modeling and Forecasting in U.S. Agriculture,* edited by G. C. Rausser. New York: North Holland, 1982.

Huber, P. W. *Liability: The Legal Revolution and Its Consequences.* New York: Basic Books, 1988.

Innes, R. "Liability Rules and Safety Regulation under Asymmetric Information." Unpublished manuscript, Department of Agricultural and Resource Economics, University of Arizona, Tucson, 1994.

Juskevich, J., and C. G. Guyer. "Bovine Growth Hormone: Human Food Safety Evaluation." *Science* August 1990: 875–84.

Klein, B., and Leffler, K. B. "The Role of Market Forces in Assuring Contractual Performance." *Journal of Political Economy* 89 (August 1981): 615–41.

Kolstad, C. D., T. S. Ulen, and G. V. Johnson. "*Ex Post* Liability for Harm vs. *Ex Ante* Safety Regulation: Substitutes or Complements?" *American Economic Review* 80 (September 1990): 888–901.

Kuchler, F., S. Lynch, K. Ralston, and L. Unnevehr. "Changing Pesticide Policies." *Choices,* 2d qtr. 1994, 15–19.

✓ Kvenberg, J. E., and D. L. Archer. "Economic Impact of Colonization Control on Foodborne Disease." *Food Technology* 41 (July 1987): 77–81, 98.

Libecap, G. D. "The Rise of the Chicago Packers and the Origins of Meat Inspection and Antitrust." *Economic Inquiry* 30 (April 1992): 242–62.

Lichtenberg, E., D. Zilberman, and K. T. Bogen. "Regulating Environmental Health Risks under Uncertainty: Groundwater Contamination in California." *Journal of Environmental Economics and Management* 17 (1989): 22–34.

Litan, R. E. "The Safety and Innovations Effects of U.S. Liability Law: The Evidence." *American Economic Review* 81 (May 1991): 59–64.

Loaharanu, P. "Cost/Benefit Aspects of Food Irradiation." *Food Technology* 48 (January 1994a): 104–8.

Loaharanu, P. "Status and Prospects of Food Irradiation." *Food Technology* 48 (May 1994b): 124–31.

Middlekauff, R. D. "Regulating the Safety of Food." *Food Technology* 43 (September 1989): 296–307.

National Research Council, Committee on Diet and Health. *Diet and Health: Implications for Reducing Chronic Disease Risk.* Washington, D.C.: National Academy Press, 1989.

National Research Council, Committee on the Nutrition Components of Food Labeling. *Nutrition Labeling: Issues and Directions for the 1990s.* Washington, D.C.: National Academy Press, 1990.

National Research Council, Committee on Pesticides in the Diets of Infants and Children. *Pesticides in the Diets of Infants and Children.* Washington, D.C.: National Academy Press, 1993.

National Research Council, Committee on Public Health Risk Assessment of Poultry Inspection Programs. *Poultry Inspection: The Basis for a Risk-Assessment Approach.* Washington, D.C.: National Academy Press, 1987.

National Research Council, Committee on the Scientific Basis of the Nation's Meat and Poultry Inspection Program. *Meat and Poultry Inspection: The Scientific Basis of the Nation's Program.* Washington, D.C.: National Academy Press, 1985.

National Research Council, Committee on Scientific and Regulatory Issues Underlying Pesticide Use Patterns and Agricultural Innovation. *Regulating Pesticides in Food: The Delaney Paradox.* Washington, D.C.: National Academy Press, 1987.

Nelson, P. "Information and Consumer Behavior." *Journal of Political Economy* 78 (1970): 311–29.

Newsome, R. "Perspectives on the Future of Food Biotechnology." *Food Technology*, September 1993, p. 106.

Nichols, A., and R. J. Zeckhauser. "The Perils of Prudence: How Conservative Risk Assessments Distort Regulation." *Regulation* 10 (November/December 1986): 11–24.

Olempska-Beer, Z. S., P. M. Kuznesof, M. DiNovi, and M. J. Smith. "Plant Biotechnology and Food Safety." *Food Technology* 47 (December 1993): 64–72.

Pierson, M. D., and D. A. Corlett, Jr., eds. *HACCP: Principles and Applications*. New York: Van Nostrand Reinhold, 1992.

Preston, W. P., A. M. McGuirk, and G. M. Jones. "Consumer Reaction to the Introduction of Bovine Somatotropin." In *Economics of Food Safety*, edited by J. A. Caswell. New York: Elsevier Science Pub. Co., 1991.

Roberts, T. "Microbial Pathogens in Raw Pork, Chicken, and Beef: Benefit Estimates for Control Using Irradiation." *American Journal of Agricultural Economics* 67 (December 1985): 957–65.

√ Roberts, T. "Human Illness Costs of Foodborne Bacteria." *American Journal of Agricultural Economics* 71 (May 1989): 468–74.

√ Roberts, T., and D. Smallwood. "Data Needs to Address Economic Issues in Food Safety." *American Journal of Agricultural Economics* 73 (August 1991): 933–42.

Rose-Ackerman, S. "Regulation and the Law of Torts." *American Economic Review* 81 (May 1991): 54–58.

Shavell, S. *Economic Analysis of Accident Law*. Cambridge: Harvard University Press, 1987.

Skully, D. "Environmental Standards and Regulations in a Global Context." In *Environmental Policies: Implications for Agricultural Trade*, edited by J. Sullivan. Washington, D.C.: U.S. Department of Agriculture, 1994.

Smallwood, D. M., and J. R. Blaylock. "Consumer Demand for Food and Food Safety: Models and Applications." In *Economics of Food Safety*, edited by J. A. Caswell. New York: Elsevier Science Pub. Co., 1991.

Smith, V. K. *Environmental Policy under Reagan's Executive Order: The Role of Benefit-Cost Analysis*. Chapel Hill: University of North Carolina Press, 1984.

Smith, V. K. "Household Production Functions and Environmental Benefit Estimation." In *Measuring the De-*

mand for Environmental Quality, edited by J. B. Braden and C. D. Kolstad. Amsterdam: North-Holland, 1991.

Stiglitz, J. E. "Imperfect Information in the Product Market." In *Handbook of Industrial Organization,* edited by R. Schmalensee and R. D. Willig. Vol. 1. Amsterdam: North-Holland Publishing Co., 1989.

U.S. Department of Agriculture, Economic Research Service. "Food Safety Issues: Modernizing Meat Inspection." *Agricultural Outlook* AO-197, June 1993, pp. 32–36.

U.S. Department of Agriculture, Office of Communications. "FSIS Pathogen Reduction/HACCP Proposal." Release No. 0077, 95, February 1, 1995.

U.S. Department of Health and Human Services. *The Surgeon General's Report on Nutrition and Health.* Washington, D.C.: Government Printing Office, 1988.

Viscusi, W. K. "Structuring an Effective Occupational Disease Policy: Victim Compensation and Risk Regulation." *Yale Journal on Regulation* 2 (1984): 53–81.

Viscusi, W. K. *Product Safety Labeling: A Federal Responsibility.* Washington, D.C.: AEI Press, 1993.

von Witzke, H., and C.-H. Hanf. "BST and International Agricultural Trade and Policy." In *Bovine Somatotropin and Emerging Issues: An Assessment,* edited by M. C. Hallberg. Boulder: Westview Press, 1992.

Winter, C. K. "Pesticide Residues and the Delaney Clause." *Food Technology* 47 (July 1993): 81–86.

Abbreviations and Acronyms

APHIS	Animal and Plant Health Inspection Service
BST	bovine somatotropin
CAST	Council for Agricultural Science and Technology
rDNA	recombinant deoxyribonucleic acid
DHHS	U.S. Department of Health and Human Services
EPA	Environmental Protection Agency
FAO	Food and Agriculture Organization of the United Nations
FDA	Food and Drug Administration
FFDCA	Federal Food, Drug, and Cosmetic Act
FIFRA	Federal Insecticide, Fungicide, and Rodenticide Act
FSIS	Food Safety Inspection Service
HACCP	Hazard Analysis Critical Control Point
NRC	National Research Council
USDA	U.S. Department of Agriculture
WHO	World Health Organization

Index

Advertising, 33

Benefit-cost analysis, 7
  current regulatory proposals, 82–84
  in Department of Agriculture, 92–93
  food irradiation, 30
  for justification of regulation, 56–60, 82
  of performance standards, 8, 69, 76, 90–91
  in setting of pesticide tolerances, 15, 16, 17
  uncertainty in, 60–61, 77
Biotechnology
  applications, 25
  BST, 28–29
  food labeling issues, 33–34
  labeling issues, 85–86
  principles of, 25, 26
  regulation of, 27–28
  safety concerns, 26–27
Bovine somatotropin, 28–29, 40, 86
BST, 40. *See* Bovine somatotropin
Bureau of Alcohol, Tobacco, and Firearms, 11–13
Bush administration, 17, 19, 32, 58

Cancer
  de minimis risk standard, 16–17
  mortality, 1–2

  negligible risk standard, 16, 17
  pesticide-related, 5–6, 35–36
Canned food, 22
Clinton administration, 17–18, 19, 21, 58, 83
Codex Alimentarius Commission, 31
Consumer behavior
  decision theory, safety considerations in, 38–39
  demand for food safety, 39–40
  firm or product safety reputation, 45–46
  in imperfect information market, 45–46
  knowledge of safety in, 52–54
  product information sources, 43
  risk preferences, 48–52, 61–63
  role of market information, 41–43
  safety knowledge, 74–77
  safety outcomes, 54–55
Costs
  design standard regulation, 65
  of diet-related health, 35
  of food contamination, 5, 34–36
  performance standard compliance, 65

safety, in perfect information equilibriums, 44–45
of supplying product safety, 49

Dairy industry, BST use in, 28–29
De minimis standard, 16–17, 63, 83, 90
Decision theory, 38–39
Delaney clause, 8, 14–18, 62, 68, 82
Design standards, 3
current regulatory approach, 86–87
destructive testing versus, 65
efficiency-inefficiency, 64, 67–68, 77
rationale, 64–66
recommendations for, 10, 91
as regulatory tool, 67–68, 73–74
versus performance standards, 63–64, 77
Diet, 35
Disease outcomes, 34–36

Egg industry, 11, 20
Environmental regulation, 18–19

Fair Packaging and Labeling Act, 33
Federal Food, Drug, and Cosmetic Act, 5
benefit-cost analysis in, 82
deficiencies of, 81
Delaney clause, 8, 14–18
food additives in, 13–14
goals of, 13
origins of, 11
Federal Insecticide, Fungicide, and Rodenticide Act, 5
benefit-cost analysis in, 82
origins of, 11
role of, 18

Fish and seafood industry
HACCP program for, 8, 22–23, 24, 25, 61, 64
regulatory history, 20–21
Food additives, 13–14
Food and Drug Administration
biotechnology regulation, 27–29
design standards, 3, 67
HACCP program, application of, 22–23, 24
labeling regulations, 33
in regulatory reform, 91–92
responsibilities, 5, 11
Food and shellfish industry
responsibility for regulation of, 11
Foreign trade
import regulation, 11
international safety standards, 31–33
Fumigation, 29–30

General Agreement on Tariffs and Trade (GATT), 32
Goals of food safety regulation, 1
efficiency as, 9
historical development, 36
recommendations for reform, 9–10, 89–90
zero risk, 44–45

HACCP. See Hazard Analysis Critical Control Points
Hazard Analysis Critical Control Points
benefit-cost analysis, 61, 88, 91
consumer concerns, 23
as design standard, 64, 87
fish and seafood industry, 8
industry concerns, 23, 87–88
industry design versus government design, 23–24

for meat and poultry industry, 22–25
performance standards, 25
principles of, 21–22, 87
rationale, 3
recommendations for, 10
research needs, 23
small firm compliance, 25
start-up costs, 3
Heart disease, 1

Import regulations, 11
Incentives, 69
Information, market
    asymmetric, 42–43
    consumer knowledge of
        safety, 52–54, 76–77
    consumer risk preferences,
        48–52, 61–63
    efficient market functioning,
        74–77
    food labeling and, 33–34
    food safety, 40, 41–43
    imperfect, 41, 42–43, 45–47,
        57
    inability to distinguish
        product quality, 46–47
    indications for regulation,
        7–8, 78, 79–80, 81
    market functioning and, 6–7
    perfect, 42, 44–45, 54
    pre- and postmarket, 6–7
    recommendations for, 10
    as regulatory tool, 66–67, 73
    safety outcomes, 54–55
International agreements, 31–33
Irradiation technology, 29–31

Labeling
    benefits of, 7
    of BST milk, 29, 86
    current performance, 8
    current regulation, 80–81
    federal regulations, 33
    new foods and technologies,
        33–34, 85–86

recommendations for, 10,
    89–90
as regulatory tool, 66–67, 73,
    77–78
responsibility for regulation
    and monitoring of, 13

Market functioning
    benefit-cost justification for
        regulation of, 56–60
    causes of inefficiency, 6
    consumer decision making,
        37
    consumer knowledge and,
        40, 41–43
    consumer knowledge of
        safety and, 52–54
    consumer risk preferences,
        48–52, 61–63
    decision theory, safety considerations in, 38–39
    demand for food safety,
        39–40
    efficiency in, 74–77, 80
    imperfect information, 45–
        46, 54–55
    indications for regulation,
        79–80, 81
    market equilibriums, 43–44
    perfect information equilibriums, 44–45
    product quality information
        in, 6–7, 41–42
    regulation versus, in delivery of safe foods, 37–38,
        55
    safety outcomes, 54–55
    supply of food safety and,
        40–41
    tort law and, 71
Meat industry
    HACCP program for, 21–25,
        64
    inspection methodology, 20
    microbial testing, 20–21,
        83–84

regulatory history, 19–21
responsibility for regulation
   and monitoring of, 11, 20
Meat Inspection Act, 11, 19
Methyl bromide, 29–30
Mortality
   cancer risk, 1–2
   food-related, 2, 34
   leading causes of death, 1
   pesticide-related cancer,
      35–36

National Marine Fisheries Ser-
   vice, 11
North American Free Trade
   Agreement (NAFTA), 32
Nutrition Labeling and Educa-
   tion Act, 33

Organic certification, 86

Performance standards, 8, 68
   advantages of, 86–88
   analytical model, 68–69
   benefit-cost analysis in, 69,
      76
   cost of compliance, 65
   deficiencies of, 65–66
   efficiency of, 68, 73, 77
   in HACCP program, 25
   recommendations for, 10,
      90–91
   versus design standards,
      63–64, 77
Pesticides
   cancer mortality, 35–36
   cancer risk, 2
   cancers caused by, 5–6
   current regulatory reform
      proposals, 83, 84–85
   Delaney clause and, 14–18
   environmental regulation,
      18–19
   food residues, detectability
      of, 15–16

food residues, legislative
   coverage of, 15
international trade and,
   32–33
recommendations for re-
   form, 90
reference dose, 14–15, 60
regulatory goals for cancer
   prevention, 2
regulatory responsibility, 5,
   11
tolerance calculations,
   14–15
Policy
   conceptual basis, 4
   current scope, 4–5
   recommendations for 1995
      farm bill, 91–93
   reform issues, 4
Political context, 59–60
Poultry industry
   HACCP program for, 21–25,
      64
   microbial testing, 83–84
   regulatory history, 19–21
   responsibility for regulation
      and monitoring of, 11, 20
Predictive modeling, of pesticide-related cancers, 5–6
Public education
   about food safety, 76
   current regulatory efforts,
      80–81, 84
   recommendations for, 10,
      89–90, 92

Rationale for government intervention
   benefit-cost analysis in,
      56–60
   design standards, 64–65
   paternalistic view, 2–3
   public education about food
      safety, 76–77
   safety research, 75, 76

Reagan administration, 58
Regulations
    benefit-cost analysis for justification of, 56–60, 82–84
    bias in development of, 8, 83
    biotechnology, 27–28
    BST, 28–29
    cancer prevention, 2
    deficiencies of, 1
    of design standards, 3
    efficiency as goal of, 9
    efficiency of, 73–78
    food irradiation, 29–31
    goals of, 9
    good qualities of, 7
    historical development, 11–16, 36
    imperfect market information and, 7, 78
    incentives in, 69
    indications for, 7–8, 78, 79–80, 81
    inefficiency of, 2–3
    labeling, 8, 33–34, 80–81
    meat inspection, 20–21
    organizational, structure for, 5, 10, 11–13
    performance standards versus design standards, 63–64
    pesticide registration for environmental assessment, 18–19
    principles of, 77–78
    public information, 66–67, 73
    recommendations for reform, 9–10, 88–91
    resource allocation, 10
    scope of, 4–5
    single-agency model, 10, 88–89
    sources of inefficiency, 9
    statutory forms, 66–69, 70, 78

    tort law, 69–73
    versus informed individual choice, 61–63, 77, 84–86
    versus market functioning in delivery of safe foods, 37–38, 55
Research
    government role, 75, 76, 80–81
    pesticide tolerances, 14–15
    recommendations for, 10, 88–90, 92
    safety labeling, 86
Risk assessment
    benefit-cost analysis and, 58
    consumer knowledge of safety in, 52–54
    de minimis standard, 16–17, 63, 83
    in HACCP, 87
    in incomplete information markets, 48–52
    individual choice versus statutory regulation, 61–63, 77, 84–86
    meaning of safety and, 38–39
    negligible risk standard, 16, 17
    pesticide-related cancer deaths, 35–36
    recommendations for regulatory reform, 90–91
    uncertainty in, 60–61

Tort law
    criticism of, 70–71
    economic theory, 70
    efficiency of, as regulatory tool, 71–72, 73, 75–76
    as regulatory system, 69–70
    statutory regulation and, 70, 72

U.S. Treasury, Department of, 11

U.S. Department of Agriculture (USDA)
  biotechnology regulation, 27
  food safety responsibilities, 5
  recommendations for, 92–93
  in single-agency model of regulation, 10
U.S. Department of Commerce, 11
U.S. Environmental Protection Agency
  Delaney clause interpretation, 16–17

pesticide registration, 19
pesticide tolerances, 14, 15
responsibilities of, 5, 11

Wholesome Meat Act, 11, 20
Wholesome Poultry Products Act, 20

Zero risk, 1, 8, 14
  benefit-cost analysis versus, 59
  in Delaney clause, 15, 16, 68
  problems of, as policy goal, 44–45
  tort law and, 72–73

About the Author

JOHN M. ANTLE is a professor in the Department of Agricultural Economics and Economics at Montana State University. During 1989–1990 he was a senior economist for the President's Council of Economic Advisers, and he contributed to two chapters in the 1990 *Economic Report of the President*.

Mr. Antle is a member of the National Research Council's Board on Agriculture and a university fellow at Resources for the Future. He was an economic consultant to research centers of the Consultative Group on International Agricultural Research, to the Rockefeller Foundation, to the National Institute for Forestry, Agriculture and Livestock Research in Mexico, and to the Organization for Economic Cooperation and Development in Paris.

Mr. Antle's research focuses on the environmental impacts of agriculture, including production, health, and environmental consequences of pesticide use in rice production in the Philippines and potato production in Ecuador, links between economic growth and the environment across low- and high-income countries, and environmental effects of pesticide use in the United States.

A NOTE ON THE BOOK

This book was edited by Ann Petty
of the American Enterprise Institute.
The figures were drawn by Hordur Karlsson.
The index was prepared by Robert Elwood.
The text was set in Palatino, a typeface
designed by the twentieth-century Swiss designer
Hermann Zapf. Coghill Composition Company of
Richmond, Virginia, set the type,
and Edwards Brothers Incorporated
of Lillington, North Carolina,
printed and bound the book,
using permanent acid-free paper.

The AEI Press is the publisher for the American Enterprise Institute for Public Policy Research, 1150 Seventeenth Street, N.W., Washington, D.C. 20036; *Christopher DeMuth,* publisher; *Dana Lane,* director; *Ann Petty,* editor; *Leigh Tripoli,* editor; *Cheryl Weissman,* editor; *Lisa Roman,* editorial assistant (rights and permissions).